MEDICAL TEXTS AND MANUSCRIPTS IN INDIAN CULTURAL HISTORY

Medical Texts and Manuscripts in Indian Cultural History

Edited by

DOMINIK WUJASTYK
ANTHONY CERULLI
KARIN PREISENDANZ

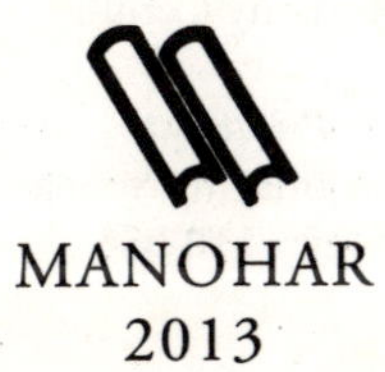

MANOHAR
2013

First published 2013

ISBN 978-93-5098-019-4

Published by
Ajay Kumar Jain *for*
Manohar Publishers & Distributors
4753/23 Ansari Road, Daryaganj
New Delhi 110 002

Design and Typesetting by
Dominik Wujastyk

Jacket design by
Anthony Cerulli

Printed at
Salasar Imaging Systems
Delhi 110 035

Contents

Preface

Medical Texts and Manuscripts in Indian Cultural History is a product of the Classical Ayurveda Text Study Group (CATS). Since its first meeting at the University of Vienna in 2003, convened by Prof. Karin Preisendanz, CATS has been bringing together scholars and practitioners of Ayurvedic medicine to discuss cutting-edge research on Indian medical history, Sanskrit medical literature, and Ayurvedic clinical practice. Past and current members of CATS have been based in Europe, India, Japan, and the United States.

The CATS group meets approximately every second year, in different international locations. At these meetings, members present new research, and consider old and new methodological and theoretical problems in Indian medical history.

A special feature of the CATS meetings was introduced at the second meeting convened by Dominik Wujastyk at University College London in 2004. While research papers are delivered in the normal way, the first two days of the meeting are set aside for reading Sanskrit medical texts in the original language together as a group. Due to the senior standing of the participants, these sessions amount to master classes in Ayurvedic textual history. Before the conference, each participant prepares a selected Sanskrit or Prakrit passage of key interest, and pre-circulates it to the group. At the conference, the group studies these texts, discussing every detail of the readings, as well as advanced technical matters of language and ancient medical theory. The participants approach these sessions with a high level of precision and a careful engagement with the grammar, syntax, textual integrity and meaning of the texts. In different ways, the members of our group are engaged in solving a host of difficult textual problems that are fundamental to the history of Indian medicine. Senior scholars commonly work in isolation, only sharing their textual endeavours through final publication. The chance to interact and share expertise during these text-reading days is unique and much appreciated by those who attend, whether as members or as guests. This particular type of literary and medical-history work is almost unknown at many universities, and CATS has been able to stimulate the introduction of the methods of advanced textual criticism and historical study in medical history at a number of university departments.

The present volume evolved out of a CATS meeting held in Coimbatore, Tamilnadu in August of 2008. The Arya Vaidya Pharmacy in Coimbatore generously supported the event, which was expertly organized by P. Ram Manohar and his staff. At that meeting CATS assembled in conjunction with the "International Grand Centennial Convention on Ayurveda and Expo." CATS convened a two-day workshop with a number of informal presentations by CATS members and invited participants. CATS then held a more formal day-long workshop on textual and manuscript studies, entitled: "The History of Medicine in India: Past and Present Theories and Practices in the Light of the Classical Textual Sources." At this pre-conference workshop twelve papers were presented, nine of which appear in the present volume.

The Coimbatore conference covered a rich selection of research. Several presenters offered innovative lines of enquiry for the historical, cultural, and textual study of Indian medicine. Of particular significance was the importance of basing research into Indian cultural history and contemporary Ayurvedic practice on the long textual and manuscript traditions of Ayurveda.

The initial two chapters of the present volume, by Cristina Pecchia and Philipp A. Maas respectively, present research from their important work on a critical edition of the Vimānasthāna of the *Carakasaṃhitā* at the Department of South Asian, Tibetan and Buddhist Studies of the University of Vienna, as part of the project series "Philosophy and Medicine in Early Classical India".[1] The chapter of Karin Preisendanz, the director of the Caraka project in Vienna, presents the first part of a substantial investigation into the history and historiography of the early phases of formal Indian philosophy. (A second part of this study is in preparation.) Dominik Wujastyk presents exciting new manuscript evidence in his chapter for establishing a cultural history of the Sanskrit medical classic, the *Suśrutasaṃhitā,* highlighting the recent discovery of a thousand-year old manuscript of the work. Anthony Cerulli offers a précis of an 18th-century Sanskrit medical allegory, the *Jīvānandanam* (*The Joy of Life*), and he argues that the text contributes novel data concerning the interplay of medicine, government, and religion in south Indian cultural history. Kenneth Zysk's chapter contains insightful information about his research in Tamilnadu on Siddha medicine and alchemy. Zysk's co-authored chapter, with Tsutomu Yamashita, reports the progress of their extensive and ongoing efforts to catalogue the extant manuscripts,

[1] Austrian Science Fund projects P17300, P19866 and P23330, preceded by the pilot project "Debate in the Context of the History of Indian Medicine," P14451.

as well as to produce a critical edition, of Jajjaṭa's very early commentary on the *Carakasaṃhitā*, the *Nirantarapada-vyākhyā*. Manoj Sankaranarayana presents a case study of the "Rescue Clyster" (*vaitaraṇavasti*) in Kerala, and he suggests this procedure illustrates one way in which Malayali vaidyas are informing their clinical practice with the Sanskrit medical classics and engaging in strategies for adapting and changing the teachings of the classical tradition in response to actual clinical experience. The chapter of P. Ram Manohar looks at the *Siddhamantra* of Keśava and, in particular, examines the text's complex contributions to the combinatoric underpinnings of Indian pharmacology.

CATS is committed to making the research of its members available as widely as possible in South Asia and throughout the world through conference presentations, workshops, and publications. Accordingly, following the 2008 Coimbatore workshop, several of the panelists agreed to publish their essays in a special issue of the *Indian Journal of the History of Science* (*IJHS*), which came out in 2009. Unfortunately, the editing of that issue was severely compromised. Errors were introduced into the essays, and titles and passages of text were re-written without consultation with the authors and sometimes against their explicit instructions. Although attempts were made to have the *IJHS* issue emended or withdrawn from circulation, in the end nothing could be done. The present volume offers these essays in the form their authors authorize, and updated with the latest research findings and interpretations. The editors of the present book have ensured that the style and presentation of the essays are consistent with the intentions of the authors.

Acknowledgements

Anthony Cerulli would like to thank the National Endowment for the Humanities for supporting his research during the writing for and production of this book. He is grateful to the Institut d'études avancées de Paris (IEA), especially Gretty M. Mirdal, Marie-Thérèse Cerf, Lisette Winkler, Florence Hulak, and Olga Spilar. IEA provided Anthony with an outstanding workspace and exceptional support during the year this book was prepared. Anthony would also like to thank the former and current provosts of Hobart and William Smith Colleges, Pat McGuire and Titilayo Ufomata respectively, for their support and encouragement to work on this volume.

Dominik Wujastyk would like to thank the Wellcome Trust for support during the writing of his contribution for this book (grant WT066401), and the Austrian Science Fund (project P23330) for support during the editing of this volume.

The editors would like to thank Prof. S. R. Sarma for first suggesting that this book might appear with Manohar Publishing, and for making the early arrangements for this to happen. Mr Ramesh Jain at Manohar has been exceptionally patient and supportive throughout the process of preparing this volume.

Special thanks go to Alexandra Böckle at the Department of South Asian, Tibetan and Buddhist Studies of the University of Vienna for her outstanding editorial assistance on this book.

Dominik Wujastyk
Anthony Cerulli
Karin Preisendanz

Contributors

Cristina Pecchia

Department of South Asian, Tibetan and Buddhist Studies, University of Vienna, Austria

Philipp A. Maas

Department of South Asian, Tibetan and Buddhist Studies, University of Vienna, Austria

Karin Preisendanz

Department of South Asian, Tibetan and Buddhist Studies, University of Vienna, Austria

Dominik Wujastyk

Department of South Asian, Tibetan and Buddhist Studies, University of Vienna, Austria

Anthony Cerulli

Department of Religious Studies and Department of Asian Languages and Cultures, Hobart and William Smith Colleges, Geneva, New York, USA

Kenneth G. Zysk

Department of Cross-cultural and Regional Studies, University of Copenhagen, Denmark

Manoj Sankaranarayana

Department of Samhita and Siddhanta, Rajiv Gandhi Ayurveda College, Mahe, Puducherry, India

Tsutomu Yamashita

Institute for Interdisciplinary Studies, Kyoto Gakuen University, Japan

P. Ram Manohar

AVP Research Foundation, Coimbatore, Tamil Nadu, India

1

Cristina Pecchia

Transmitting the *Carakasaṃhitā*: Notes for a History of the Tradition

The theorist of textual criticism, Giorgio Pasquali, remarked that the best editor of an ancient work that is transmitted, for instance, in medieval manuscripts, will be the one who knows the work, its language, its time and the language of its times, and, at the same time, the time in which the manuscripts were produced.[1] This reflection is the reason

The present research was funded by the Austrian Science Fund (FWF) within the research project P19866, *Philosophy and Medicine in Early Classical India II*, based at the University of Vienna, under the direction of Karin Preisendanz, with Philipp A. Maas and the present writer as collaborators. My gratitude goes to the Arya Vaidya Pharmacy for its generous invitation to the Conference "The History of Medicine in India: Past and Present Theories and Practices in the Light of the Classical Textual Sources," held in Coimbatore, 22 August 2008, where a previous version of the present paper was read.

[1]Paraphrase of Pasquali 1952: 123: "Il miglior critico di un testo greco di tradizione bizantina sarà quello che, oltre a essere un perfetto grecista, sia anche perfetto bizantinista. Il miglior editore di un autore latino trasmesso in codici medievali o postmedievali sarà colui che, quanto il suo autore e la sua lingua e i suoi tempi e la lingua dei suoi tempi, altrettanto bene conosca il Medioevo o l'umanesimo." Pasquali adds that such an editor is an ideal that nobody can perfectly embody, but everyone should strive to come close to it ("Un critico siffatto è un ideale che

why the history of the work's tradition is a subject of study for those who approach a work from the point of view of textual criticism. Both manuscript and printed books are one of the main subjects of study for the history of a work's tradition, and even more relevant in connection with the paucity of other primary sources, namely archive documents like private papers, account books and business correspondence, as well as sources like histories of libraries and manuscript collections. Raising the issue of the work's transmission is also, of necessity, an exploration in the history of education and scholarship, in the wider intellectual and cultural history of specific geographical areas, groups of persons and institutions in South Asia.[2]

The considerations that I shall present concern the history of the transmission of the *Carakasaṃhitā* (henceforth *CS*), more in particular the *Vimānasthāna*, which is the subject of a critical edition under preparation at the University of Vienna.[3] I shall analyse philological activities, seats of learning, patronage structures, and so on. The object of analysis and interpretation will be limited to one type of production of the textual transmission, namely the manuscript books.[4] I leave aside at present the category of printed books, which also requires observations concerning the history of printing in India and therefore a partially differ-

---

nessuno può incarnare in sé perfettamente, ma al quale ognuno ha il dovere di cercare di avvicinarsi.").

[2] A classic work that exposes the processes by which Greek and Latin literature have been preserved and transmitted is Reynolds and Wilson 1991.

[3] See preliminary note, p. 1 above.

[4] The word "manuscript book" is used with reference to a set of sheets of paper, or other material, that is a text-bearer. No reference is made to the aspect of binding. Throughout the present paper, the word "manuscript" will be freely used in the sense of "manuscript book."

ent range of information and methods of analysis.[5] Furthermore, I shall address the question of research strategies, also pointing out problems and limits in the sources from which interpretations arise.

Manuscript books as sources for the history of a textual tradition

Manuscript books bear information on different levels, according to "their bifunctional role," namely as both archaeological object, or "container," and as intellectual message, or textual "content".[6] When we consider a manuscript as a container, we examine it from a codicological[7] and paleographical point of view; that is to say, we examine the manuscript from the point of view of its materiality and graphical representation of the text, including scripts, signs, seals, and so on. When we investigate the content of a manuscript, we analyse the text that is contained in it, also including scribal colophons, which can be a particularly precious source.[8] In the case of the *CS*, they are not always present.

---

[5]This will be the subject of a future publication, that will address the spatial-temporal coordinates in which the data of the transmission of the work should be placed.

[6]See Scherrer-Schaub and Bonani 2002: 186.

[7]In the field of indological studies, the discipline of the study of manuscripts as cultural artifacts is called, for some reason, "manuscriptology," using a neologism (maybe on the basis of the German word Handschriftenkunde?), instead of "codicology," which is the existing current designation. Muzerelle has fixed the technical terminology of codicology in his 1985 major publication; its language is French, which, for historical reasons, is one of the main vehicular languages of the discipline. Based on Muzerelle's work, a codicological vocabulary is being established in other languages.

[8]Colophons in medieval European texts have long been a separate subject of study. This kind of analysis is also being developed in the field of Tibetan studies; more recently, see Clemente 2007. With regard to manuscripts containing Sanskrit texts, Banerjee 1987 provides some

This fact is also a result of the fragmentation of the work in individual *sthānas*, which, especially if they originally belonged to the wider framework of the *Saṃhitā*, were not closed by the copyist by means of a colophon. The scanty number of scribal colophons is also the reason why the precise date and place of production of many manuscripts remain unknown.

Manuscript books, furthermore, have spatial-temporal coordinates, which reveal information about the time and contexts in which they were produced, acquired, used, exchanged, preserved, etc., and which allow some inferences regarding, for instance, how the work circulated and was perceived. The information we can gather from these investigations goes under four main categories: time, places, agents and modalities of the transmission.

Only some reflections deriving from this very wide spectrum of data and observations will be exposed in the following.

The *Carakasaṃhitā* as a composite work[9]

At present, 236 manuscripts containing the *CS* are known. Most of them are known through direct record in catalogues and hand-lists, and some through their being mentioned by editors of printed books of the *CS*. Among them, forty-nine copies of manuscripts containing the *Vimānasthāna* are available for the critical edition under preparation. These copies are in different materials, namely paper

---

examples and related reflections. The same author repeats most of them, with slight changes, in his 1991 article.

[9]In the following, I will refer to material that Karin Preisendanz, Ernst Prets and Philipp A. Maas collected for the research project P17300, *Philosophy and Medicine in Early Classical India I*, funded by the Austrian Science Fund (FWF); Yasutaka Muroya photographed one manuscript on behalf of the same project.

copies, microfilms and digital copies; another five manuscripts kept in the Anup Sanskrit Library at Bikaner could be only collated on the spot. About ten manuscripts that are kept in public and private libraries in India could not be used so far. The original manuscript books are written on paper and in different scripts, namely Devanāgarī, Bengali, Śāradā and Kannaḍa.

A first remark regarding these data is that the text of the *Vimānasthāna* is only contained in a few manuscripts. In fact, only a minority of the manuscripts containing the *CS* includes the entire work, while many manuscripts only contain one or more *sthāna*s. This shows that the *CS*, at least at a certain point of its history, also circulated as a composite work, as a set of texts, each *sthāna* being a distinct unit. In fact, we have manuscript books that contain individual *sthāna*s, but sometimes their foliation or pagination suggests that they belonged to a larger book, because the first folio does not bear the number one. It is likely that the work was fragmented in connection with either a "preservation policy," or a "market policy," or just on practical grounds. Furthermore, the undoubted fact that some books bear two foliations, namely one for the entire book and one for each individual *sthāna*, indicates that the work was perceived as a set of independent parts. This way of perceiving the work facilitated and legitimized its circulation by way of individual *sthāna*s.

Time of the manuscript transmission: the documented period

We have a huge chronological gap between the composition of the *Vimānasthāna*, which approximately goes back to the second century CE, and the oldest dated available manuscript, Alipur, Bhogilal Leherchand Institute of Indology

45283, which was copied in 1592. The manuscripts that have no date, which are approximately 50%, do not present signs of considerable antiquity. Neither the material, nor the types of scripts indicate that the witnesses might be older than the 16th century. The most recent manuscripts, on the contrary, are unusually late. Even though they are not dated, they may be assigned to the beginning of the 20th century. Two of these manuscripts are preserved in Jamnagar, at the Gujarat Ayurved University Library,[10] and share some similarities with another manuscript that is dated 1st November 1945.[11] Therefore, the directly documented history of the manuscript transmission of the *Vimānasthāna* spans more than three centuries and begins at the very end of the 16th century. Other *sthāna*s have a different history. The *Cikitsāsthāna*, in particular, is attested in a manuscript kept in Kathmandu, the National Archives, Durbar Library 1-1648, dated 1183 CE, written in old Devanāgarī on palm leaf.

The available manuscripts of the *Vimānasthāna* presuppose a long chain of copies, of which just the last part is extant. The critical reconstruction of the text has thus to rely on witnesses that belong to a much later historical period and are actually the result of processes by which the text was molded over the centuries. The conditions of the manuscript tradition suggest that, in the course of its history, no dramatic break occurred, but different lines of transmission crystallized. The fact that books containing the entire *CS*, including the *Vimānasthāna*, appear at the end of the sixteenth century firstly indicates that the work was copied several times in that century; secondly, that manuscripts were relatively well kept. In fact, manuscript

[10] They are the manuscripts GAS 103 and GAS 118.

[11] Jamnagar, Gujarat Ayurved University Library, GAS 113.

books of the *Vimānasthāna* consistently appear in a period in which courtly or state institutions support, control and organize the intellectual inheritance of their territory, as the existence of a preservation policy shows.

It would be difficult to place a substantial appearing of manuscripts of the entire *CS* in a period different from that in which textual foundations of knowledge-systems are not only recuperated with new textual and stylistic attention, but they are also seen for the first time as *part* (indeed the fundamental centre) of a tradition from which the idea of innovation cannot be dissociated.[12]

As stated by Sheldon Pollock, the two centuries from about 1550 to 1750 "witnessed a flowering of scholarship, [...] including a degree of attentiveness to the historicity of intellectual life previously unexampled."[13] Furthermore, a "revitalized interest in textual foundations seems to be a hallmark of the early-modern knowledge-systems."[14]

The places of the transmission

The present provenance of the manuscripts of the *CS*, namely the public or private libraries and collections in which the manuscripts are found now (see Appendix, p. 23), can offer an approximate indication of the area of their primary provenance. This consideration also implies that there is no reason why the manuscript copies of a

---

[12]In the present sentence, I have paraphrased, *mutatis mutandis*, a passage in Antonelli 1985: 145, in which the author shows the link between tradition, interpretation and textual criticism in the culture of medieval Europe by referring to some types of manuals on textual criticism, written in twelfth-century Rome. It is worth noting that the problematic of language and science, which is exposed by Pollock 2007 (especially pp. 209–15) with reference to early-modern India, is also a major subject in thirteenth-century medieval Europe.

[13]Pollock 2007: 204. See also Pollock 2001.

[14]Pollock 2002: 434.

work that are preserved in a library should be related to each other in terms of genealogy.[15] The actual origin of a manuscript remains to be inferred by means of the manuscript itself, namely by means of the information that can be gathered from the manuscript both as archaeological object and textual content, especially when other primary sources for the book-history are missing.

The provenance of the *Vimānasthāna* manuscripts first of all reveals that this text is almost absent in the libraries of South India, except for a very recent and incomplete copy that is kept at the Oriental Research Institute of Mysore. The type of ink, paper and script, a very cursive Kannaḍa, seems to suggest that the copy was most probably written in the 20th century. Furthermore, the presence of some forms of paratext, like chapter titles, indicates that it is not a modern transcription of an older manuscript, or, at least, certainly not only a transcription. Two other fragments of the *CS*, which, however, do not contain the *Vimānasthāna*, are kept in Madras: one at the Archaeological Department (no. 183) and another at the Government Oriental Manuscript Library (no. 13090). Except for these very fragmentary copies from Madras and Mysore, the most "Southern," so to say, manuscripts of the *Vimānasthāna*, but also of the *CS*, come from the Asiatic Society of Bombay (dated śaka 1786, i.e., 1864 CE) and from the Bhandarkar Oriental Research Institute and the Ānandāśrama in Pune. This fact indicates that at a certain point, in South India, the *CS*'s popularity declined. Most likely, the dominance of another work belonging to the same discipline caused a decrease in the production of new copies, to such an extent that the number of circulating manuscripts was not sufficient to guarantee the preservation of the work.

---

[15] See Pasquali 1952: 39, n. 2.

By looking at the list of the extant manuscripts containing the *Vimānasthāna* (see Appendix, p. 23), their places of provenance are distributed over two main geographical areas, namely Bengal and North-West India. They roughly correspond to the areas of the Kaśmīri recension and the Eastern recension, namely the two main versions of the text that can be identified through the textual critical work. Both versions, however, circulated in the whole northern area. For some textual features, namely variant readings and typology of scribal errors, suggest that a few manuscripts, which are written in Devanāgarī and preserved in libraries of North-West India, derive from a Bengali version. In this regard, we can suppose a few scenarios: manuscripts that had a specific version of the text and were written in Bengali script were copied in Devanāgarī and eventually arrived in North-West manuscript collections. Another possibility is that they migrated towards North-West India, where they were either faithfully copied in Devanāgarī, or, by conflation, partially incorporated in a local extant version of the text. We have also to assume the opposite direction of migration, because two manuscripts in Bengali script show very strong features of the Kaśmīri recension, mixed with those of the Eastern recension; they are the Varanasi manuscript, Sarasvati Bhavan Library 44842, and the Calcutta manuscript, Asiatic Society G 2503/1.

Centres of manuscript book collections: modern India

It is reasonable to assume that the written transmission of the *Vimānasthāna* and *CS* in South India had already broken up before the middle of the 19th century, when a number of scholars went in search of manuscripts in different areas of the Indian subcontinent, collecting the manuscripts and writing *Reports* and *Notices* on their activity. Their main impulse was the wish to take possession of the Indian knowledge, which was still deposited in the form of manuscript books, not in printed books.[16] This wish was also inspired by "a purely utilitarian principle," as we can read in the following statement by the Major-General H. M. Durand:[17]

> I am not in favour of devoting exorbitant sums to the sentimental nurture of Sanskrit or Arabic literature; but, so long as both these languages remain what they are, — the radical sources of enormous spiritual influence on millions under our rule, — I am averse, even from a purely utilitarian principle, to neglect their ancient utterances; for they remain a living power among those millions.

The search continued for many years and in large areas, because it became clear that various sources had to be reached, from private collections to libraries connected to different cultural institutions.

A large quantity of manuscript books, which were the result of this search, constituted the main, or even the first fund of public repositories of manuscripts.[18] In Calcutta, for instance, "[t]he collection of Ayurvedic manuscripts of the Asiatic Society can be traced as early as 1871 CE, when the 'Notices of Sanskrit Manuscripts, Vol. I' was published by Sir Rājendralāla Mitra."[19] The five manuscripts contain-

---

[16]The concern for the loss of "Indian" knowledge appeared also more recently, in terms of loss of a system of knowledge, in Vatsyayan 2006: 56 in particular.

[17]"Minute by Major-General the Hon'ble Sir H. M. Durand, C.B., K.C.S.I., — dated Simla, the 13th August 1868," in Gough 1878: 8. I would like to thank Thomas Kintaert (University of Vienna), who provided me with this book.

[18]See Sarma 2001: 414 f., and Patel and Kumar 2001: 10.

[19]Bandury and Gupta 2006: viii.

ing the *CS* that are kept at the Bhandarkar Oriental Research Institute, Pune, were collected by R. G. Bhandarkar during the years 1882–1883[20] and by Abaji Vishnu Kathavate during the years 1891–1895.[21] The collection at the Gujarat Ayurved University Library in Jamnagar, with 27 manuscripts of the *CS*, was most likely enlarged in connection with the edition and translation of the *CS* made by the Shree Gulabkunverba Ayurvedic Society, whose result was the work's publication in 1949, in Jamnagar.[22] Some of the Jamnagar manuscripts are twentieth-century transcriptions of older manuscripts. In the case of the *Vimānasthāna*, one manuscript was certainly directly copied from a manuscript that is now kept in Bikaner and another one was most probably copied also collating the same Bikaner manuscript.[23] The Gulabkunverba Ayurvedic Society represents a recent case of "courtly" patronage. For patron of the Society was His Highness Namdar Maharaja Jam Saheb Shree and president of the Society was Her Highness Maharani Shree Gulabkunverba Sahiba of Nawanagar.

Centres of manuscript book collections: early-modern North-West India

Large manuscript collections were established in court libraries of North-West medieval India.[24] They normally contained books that were an exclusive product made for the patron, i.e., the Mahārājas' families, who were interested in collecting works belonging to various fields of knowl-

[20] Bhandarkar 1884: 83.

[21] Kathavate 1901.

[22] The book contains the edition of the Sanskrit text and translation in Hindi, Gujarati and English. The names of the members of the editorial board are listed at pp. 1–2 of the first volume.

[23] See Pecchia 2010, §§ 4.3 and 4.4.

[24] See Patel and Kumar 2001: 5–7.

edge as part of their larger enterprise of collecting the contents of the intellectual culture produced in their kingdoms. Bikaner and Jaipur, for example, were and still are great repositories of manuscript books. Ayurveda was an important knowledge-system of the time, because each manuscript collection contains many Ayurvedic works.

Jaipur The Mahārājas of Jaipur had an active role as "cultural entrepreneurs".[25] Their collection of manuscripts and paintings was constantly enlarged by acquisition and production. They also had a refined system of maintenance, preservation and classification of manuscripts.[26] Surely, their library (*pothīkhānā*) testifies to their interest in Ayurveda and other systems of medical knowledge.[27] Mirza Rājā Jay Singh (1621–1667)[28] was the first ruler who properly organized the collection of manuscripts he had inherited from his forefathers. His son Ram Singh I (1667–1689)[29] continued the family tradition concerning the increase of the manuscript production and the organization of the library. Ram Singh I also used to put on his manuscripts his own seal, which has, from the top to the bottom, *rāma*, a

[25]For information about the Mahārājas' dynasty, their literary activity and heritage, see the first section, "Literary Heritage of the Rulers of Amber and Jaipur," in Bahura 1976.

[26]See Bahura 1976: 15–20 (first section). Bahura also reports, "it had been a practice among the princes and the potentates to store such objects [i.e., manuscripts and paintings] close by their bedrooms." (*ibidem*, p. 15).

[27]See Bahura 1976: 3–130 (second section "An Index to the register of manuscripts in the Pothikhana of Jaipur – (i) Khas-mohor"), in which Bahura provides an alphabetical Index of the Sanskrit Works according to the Register of Manuscripts.

[28]See Bahura 1976: 15 and 37–42 (first section). For the genealogy of the rulers of Amber and Jaipur and their reigns, see Bahura 1976: 11.

[29]See Bahura 1976: 11, 16 and 42–45 (first section).

lion and the case-ending *sya*; at the top, split in two parts, the date 1718 (*vikrama saṃvat*), that is 1661 CE.[30]

Based on Ram Singh I's seal, a *terminus ante quem* can be assigned to the undated manuscript Maharaja Sawai Man Singh II Museum 2068, in Jaipur. We may conventionally assume that the date before which the manuscript must have been written is 1690 CE, namely after the death of Ram Singh I, because we do not have any precise information regarding the span of time in which the seal was actually used. However, it seems to be unusual that Ram Singh I used for many years a dated seal of the time in which he was not yet a Mahārāja.

The next generations of Mahārājas maintained and enlarged the library, in which medical texts had a conspicuous role. Sawai Pratap Singh (1778–1803)[31] is also said to have composed an Ayurvedic work, the *Amṛtasāgar* ("Ocean of Nectar," 1864), even though, most likely, somebody else composed it for him.[32]

An interesting aspect of these early Mahārājas of Amber and Jaipur is their contact with the city of Kāśī. Mirza Rājā Jay Singh, in fact, founded a college in Kāśī, in which also his son, the future Ram Singh I, studied. Furthermore, both rulers were associated with pandits and poets who lived in Kāśī; hence the implication that they held Sanskrit literat-

[30]See Bahura 1976: 16 (first section) and Plate VI.b. This date shows that he began organizing his library when he was not yet the ruler of Amber (the capital was moved to Jaipur by Sawai Jai Singh II, reign 1699–1743).

[31]The reign is taken from Bahura 1976: 11. The date that is given in Stark 2007: 409, seems to put together Sawai Prithivi Singh's and Sawai Pratap Singh's reign.

[32]See Bahura 1976: 80 (first section), Stark 2007: 409, and Meulenbeld 1999–2002: IIA, 341 *et passim*.

ure and language in high esteem.[33] This fact gives evidence of a vital cultural exchange between Rajasthan and Eastern India (with special reference to the cultural centre of Kāśī) and can be related, and supposed to be the cause of, the exchange that is observed in the textual tradition of the *Vimānasthāna* (see above, p. 7 "The places of the transmission").

Another interesting aspect of the early Mahārājas of Amber and Jaipur is their contact with the Bikaner ruling family. Ram Singh I, in particular, was Anup Singh's "friend and fellow bibliophile" and they also exchanged manuscripts.[34]

Bikaner Bikaner is the place in which the highest number of manuscripts containing the *CS* or sections of it is preserved. The city has at present two libraries, in which manuscripts are kept: the Rajasthan Oriental Research Institute of Bikaner, where the Shree Motichand Khajanchi Collection is preserved, with three manuscripts of the *CS*, and the Anup Sanskrit Library, which has 33 manuscripts of the *CS*, although only two of them contain the complete work. The Anup Sanskrit Library houses the collection of manuscripts assembled by Anup Singh (also spelt "Anūpasiṃha," reign 1669 to 1698)[35] and the following Mahārājas of Bikaner. One important feature of this library is that it contains many manuscripts that come from the Deccan. There was, in fact, "a vast influx of scientific texts from the South into Rājasthān"[36] when Anup Singh was campaign-

[33]Bahura 1976: 38 and 44 (first section), and Pingree 1997: 103.

[34]See Bahura 1976: 44 (first section) and Pingree 1997, *ibidem*.

[35]See Pingree 1997: 91. See Pingree 1997: 91–103 for a survey of Anup Singh's activity as collector of manuscripts, with special reference to those of *jyotiṣa* texts.

[36]Pingree 1997: 103.

ing in the Deccan together with Aurangzīb's army.[37] As far as the *CS* is concerned, however, the Rajasthan copies do not reveal any particular influence or direct provenance from traditions different from those transmitted by other northern copies.

Bikaner was most probably a centre in which Ayurvedic manuscripts were also collected from other areas. For a manuscript in Śāradā script, which is now in the collection of the Bhandarkar Oriental Research Institute, Pune, was acquired in Bikaner by Georg Bühler during his search of Sanskrit manuscripts in 1875–1876.[38] However, because of its script and the vertical format of its folios, it is reasonable to assume that the manuscript was produced in Kaśmīr.

Patrons and copyists of the *Vimānasthāna*: some cases

Patronage

As the manuscript collections in the libraries show, the professional hand-written production of books was a flourishing activity in 17th–18th century India.[39] This activity was sponsored, or mainly sponsored, by cultural and political institutions, which, aiming at preserving, transmitting and developing different knowledge-systems, also set up or supported the book production. The presence of a generous patronage involved the presence of professionals of writing (*lekhaka*); for they can only exist if a significant category of people who commission manuscripts exists. When

[37] Pingree 1997: 99.

[38] The manuscript corresponds to no. 555 of the 1875–76 list by Bühler (1877: xxxvi) and belongs to the Deccan College Collection. It was catalogued by Sharma (1939: p. 80, #65). The manuscript was copied in 1688 CE.

[39] For the general remarks contained in the following paragraphs, I mainly consulted Bühler 1960, in which the production of the European fifteenth-century book is under examination.

such a category of professionals of writing is established, then it is available on the market of the book production and can be employed by wealthy people who want to have their own library.

Somebody who commissioned a manuscript book will not necessarily make use of it, but he, or she, may just want to possess a copy of a specific work. Therefore, the exterior and physical conditions of the manuscripts not only provide some quite accurate information about the kind of copyist who produced them, but also, if this is the case, about the patronage that supported their production. Some manuscripts of the *Vimānasthāna*, which are in very good material conditions, show that they were not intensively used, or even not used at all. This fact suggests that the main purpose of the persons who commissioned the copies was simply the possession and/or preservation of the work itself. If this is typical of royal patrons, it must have been true also for other types of wealthy patrons, who organize and maintain large libraries, because royal patrons commissioned only a minority of the extant manuscripts.

Among other possible sources of patronage for the *CS*, we should take into account also the specific category of physicians. They might have been interested in commissioning copies of the work on practical grounds, namely in order to use it as a reference book in the medical practice and in the teaching activity, both for themselves and for their students.

Professionals of writing

The task of professional copyists consisted in reading and copying the text of their exemplar; it was distinct from the act of understanding the text's content. As readings in the manuscripts show again and again, professional copyists were often not much conversant with the language of the text they were copying. This fact allows us to infer that a low level of linguistic competence was not an obstacle to the profession. Furthermore, the act of writing was not an elite intellectual activity in itself, but also "just a job." Conversely, Sanskrit was deliberately administered as an elite language. The competence in writing is very specific, but this does not *per se* imply that writing is an exclusive activity of the intellectual elite. The activity of writing can certainly be the distinctive feature of an elite group, but the one that is chiefly defined by the fact that it exists in a context of illiteracy.

The manuscripts of the *Vimānasthāna* are, in most of the cases, produced by professional copyists. The typical feature of their work is that the general exterior aspect of the manuscript looks nice and neat and its script regular, with no particular inclination and with no unbalanced distribution of letters in the line; however, the manuscript may easily bear an inaccurate text.

The copyist of the Pune manuscript Ānandāśrama 1546 (dated 1799), for example, explicitly states the limits of his task, which he duly performed. For he writes in the colophon a *śloka* that is a copyists' standard phrase:[40]

> *yādṛśaṃ pustakaṃ dṛṣṭvā tādṛśaṃ likhitaṃ mayā*
> *yadi śuddham aśuddhaṃ vā mama doṣo na vidyate*
> As I read the book, so I have written it.
> If it is correct or incorrect, it is not my fault.

The copyist clearly distinguishes between the material and textual aspects of the book. By means of the former aspect, a

[40]See Filliozat 1941: xviii, Banerjee 1987: 76 and 1991: 10, for similar sentences in other Indian manuscript books and Bühler 1960: 21 for Medieval European manuscript books.

manuscript serves its function of exemplar and is the object of the copying activity (*likhitaṃ*). The latter aspect does not belong to that activity; this is the reason why the copyist is not responsible for the correctness of the text, about which, however, he raises doubts.[41]

An extreme case of the combination of nice appearance and inaccurate text, as well as of the copyist's awareness of the specificity of copying, is the manuscript Bikaner, Rajasthan Oriental Research Institute (RORI) 1566, in Devanāgarī, dated 1797 CE. In the colophon, the copyist says his name, Tṛpāṭhī Raghunātha, and place of origin, Saravāḍa,[42] which might be the modern Sarwar, near Ajmer.[43] On the basis of the colophons of these two Bikaner manuscripts, we can say that, at the end of the 18th century, a place called Saravāḍa was a centre of the MS production and the *Carakasaṃhitā* was one of the texts that were commissioned there. Its copyist just wrote what he could read in his exemplar, sometimes producing sequences of letters that do not make any sense. Analysing a sample section of the *Vimānasthāna*, namely 8.1–14, the manuscript has a number of individual erroneous readings that corresponds to 27% of the text. The appearance of the folios, on the contrary, is good and the style of writing very clear and

[41] Banerjee's interpretation of the copyist's intent in this *śloka* differs from the one I exposed. He says: "Here the copyist frankly admits that he is not always competent enough to discriminate between what is correct (*śuddha*) and what is incorrect (*aśuddha*) in the MSS. It appears that it was not possible for one to judge the correctness of the language of a MS with the content of which he was not always conversant." (Banerjee 1991: 10).

[42] *saṃvat 1854 [.. .ke] vaiśāṣaśuklapaṃcamī somabāre liṣitaṃ | tṛpāṭhī raghunātha saravāḍamadhye ||*

[43] From the same place another copyist comes: Pujārīgopālaḥ, who wrote the MS preserved in Bikaner, Rajasthan Oriental Research Institute, no. 1564 (1799/1800 CE), containing the *Cikitsāsthāna* only.

regular. About the reasons why a manuscript bears a text with so many errors, it can be assumed that the copyist not only made orthographical errors, as it is usual, but he also read an exemplar that must have been very bad in terms of text and also physical conditions. For it is clear from the variant readings that the copyist interpreted sequences of *akṣaras* as mere visual objects, and not as units bearing a meaning, to such an extent that it is plausible to assume that he was forced to do so from the bad quality of what he could read in his exemplar. This "bad" exemplar was most likely the final result of a long sequence of reproductions, in which involuntary orthographical errors induced by features of the handwriting were multiplied by the features of a script that represented a writing system different from the one adopted by the copyist. Some readings in the Bikaner manuscript can be explained, in fact, as the result of a sequence of errors in reading and writing that developed from one act of copying to the other. Yet, one can recognize some traces of a previous exemplar that must have been written in a kind of Devanāgarī with *pṛṣṭhamātrā* "e," or in a Bengali script, in which this kind of "e" is the most common.

This Bikaner manuscript also evidences the conditions in which some representatives of the *CS* tradition were at the end of the 18th century. Moreover, considering the textual meaning one can gain from this copy, it is evident that the actual content of the manuscript was not a primary factor for the one who commissioned it. We may thus infer that he wanted to have a copy of the work in his personal library, but not necessarily in order to consult it. About the reasons why the exemplar of this Bikaner manuscript was valuable enough to be copied, one can speculate that its provenance made it valuable, or its being a unique copy of the *CS* in the area in which it was copied. It is highly probable indeed that the commission was due to the material conditions of the book, which had already reached a critical stage. Copying the manuscript was the only way to save it.[44] Indeed, copying also had the specific function of reproducing an existing manuscript book, whose value was the text as such, no matter what the letter of the text of the work was.

Semi-professional copyists

A second category of copyists is that of the semi-professional copyists. In the case of Ayurvedic works, we can assume two main types: 1) physicians who were not scholars, who copied the text to have it as a reference book at their disposal, and 2) students, who copied the work in order to study it, or for their teacher. A case in point seems to be the manuscript Pune, Bhandarkar Oriental Research Institute, no. 925 of the 1891-95 list by Kathavate.

Learned copyists: professionals and copyists for themselves

Because writing was also a competence of learned people, we may find copyists for whom writing is not exclusively, or not at all, a work occupation. They represent the category of the "learned" copyists, who may transcribe books as professionals, but also as part of their wider intellectual activity. In fact, learned copyists can be copyists "for themselves," who copy texts for their own use. With regard to Ayurvedic works, they may typically be scholar-physicians, who also copied texts to make them available to their students. The work of copyists for themselves can be sometimes recognized through the mere appearance of

[44] See Colas 1999: 31.

the book. For these copyists can neglect the formal aspects of the books: because they were much poorer in means than the institutions, they might transcribe the text they copied just for their own use on a cheap material, with a bad quality ink and, especially, with an irregular and inaccurate way of writing.[45] Furthermore, copyists for themselves employed the margins as space to note down personal comments as well as paraphrases and quotations from other works.[46]

An important feature of learned copyists and copyists for themselves is that they may easily manipulate the letter of what they read in their exemplar, either according to other copies available to them or according to their own understanding, going through aware or unaware processes, from deliberate alterations to Freudian slips.[47] For these kinds of copyists the priority is the manuscript as a bearer of content, and not as a material object. They also show that the tradition of the work is alive, that there are scholars who study the work.

An example of a copy made (also) for personal use is most probably Varanasi, Sarasvati Bhavan Library 108685, which is written in a very cursive Bengali script. The manuscript, which contains many glosses written in the margins, was evidently a copy used to study the work, making comments here and there on the folios, without paying attention to the way in which the manuscript would appear afterwards. This copy bears striking textual similarities to the manuscript Varanasi, Sarasvati Bhavan Library

[45]This description of a type of learned copyist is a paraphrase from Pasquali 1952: 32, n. 1.

[46]It cannot be excluded that marginal notes contain information deriving from the oral tradition.

[47]Timpanaro (1975) offers interesting considerations of the subject of the Freudian slip as applied to textual criticism.

108824, which belonged to Gaṅgādhara, the author of the *CS*'s commentary *Jalpakalpataru* and first editor of the *CS*; for his edition of the *Sūtrasthāna* of the *CS* appeared in 1868, in Bengali script, at the Samvadajnanaratnakar Press (Calcutta). The next edition, which contained the entire *CS* together with Gaṅgādhara's *Jalpakalpataru* was published by Dharanidhar Ray Kaviraj and printed by Pramadabhanjana Press, in Bahrampur, Saidabad, in 1878/79 (*saṃvat* 1935).[48]

Conclusion

Even though there are so many gaps in our knowledge of the history of the *CS*'s manuscript tradition, certain patterns are discernible and point to a diversified, but unbroken, textual tradition. Through the different lines of transmission that are witnessed by the genealogical relationships among manuscripts, we still have traces of the interpretative acts that were performed in the course of the transmission and traces of the changes in the perception of the text that scholarship and education brought about. The reproduction of manuscripts by professional copyists, because of the patronage that they presuppose, shows that Ayurveda was not only a practice, an applied knowledge, with a set of efficacious preparations, but also represented a specific system of knowledge, with a body of works in which this knowledge is contained, also including foundational works. The *CS* is an instance of this kind of works, because it has a bidirectional function: it has a content that bears a specific scientific value and, at the same time, it is an authoritative representative of a specific knowledge-system, systematized by somebody called Caraka. The foundational role of the *CS*, together with the awareness of the existence of a specific medical system, was uninterrupted over centuries,

[48]See Meulenbeld 1999–2002: IB, 3.

and so was the transmission of the work. One may speculate about the reasons of the awareness of the specificity of one's own tradition. One of the possible reasons is that it also developed because of the contemporaneous presence, in the same place, of other medical traditions, with regard to North-West India, especially the Unani system.

Appendix

List of the extant manuscripts available to the project (see preliminary note, p. 1 and footnote 9) containing the *Vimānasthāna*

1. Ahmedabad, B. J. Institute of Learning and Research 758
2. Alipur, Bhogilal Leherchand Institute of Indology 45283
3. Alipur, Bhogilal Leherchand Institute of Indology 5527
4. Alwar, Rajasthan Oriental Research Institute 2498
5. Baroda, Oriental Institute 12489
6. Baroda, Oriental Institute, Ayurveda 8–52
7. Bikaner, Rajasthan Oriental Research Institute 1566
8. Bikaner, Anup Sanskrit Library 124
9. Bikaner, Anup Sanskrit Library 125
10. Bikaner, Anup Sanskrit Library 134
11. Bikaner, Anup Sanskrit Library 135
12. Bikaner, Anup Sanskrit Library 136
13. Bombay, Asiatic Society 172
14. Calcutta, National Library RDS 101
15. Calcutta, Library of Calcutta Sanskrit College 23
16. Calcutta, Library of Calcutta Sanskrit College 24
17. Calcutta, Asiatic Society G 4474/3
18. Calcutta, Asiatic Society G 2503/1
19. Calcutta, Asiatic Society G 4391
20. Cambridge, Trinity College Library R 15.85
21. Chandigarh, Lal Chand Research Library 2315
22. Ilāhābad, G. Jha Kendriya Sanskrit Vidyapeetha 25398
23. Ilāhābad, G. Jha Kendriya Sanskrit Vidyapeetha 8783/87
24. Ilāhābad, G. Jha Kendriya Sanskrit Vidyapeetha 37089
25. Jaipur, Maharaja Sawai Man Singh II Museum 2068
26. Jaipur, Maharaja Sawai Man Singh II Museum 2069

27. Jaipur, Maharaja Sawai Man Singh II Museum 2561
28. Jammu, Raghunath Temple Library 3266
29. Jammu, Raghunath Temple Library 3209
30. Jammu, Raghunath Temple Library 3330
31. Jamnagar, Gujarat Ayurved University Library GAS 103
32. Jamnagar, Gujarat Ayurved University Library GAS 118
33. Jamnagar, Gujarat Ayurved University Library GAS 96/2
34. Jamnagar, Gujarat Ayurved University Library GAS 119
35. Koṭa, Rajasthan Oriental Research Institute 1563
36. Kathmandu, Nepal German Manuscript Preservation Project E-40553
37. London, Indian Office Library, Sanskrit 335
38. London, Indian Office Library, Sanskrit 881
39. London, Indian Office Library, Sanskrit 1445b
40. Mysore, Oriental Research Institute 902 (107,6)
41. Pune, Bhandarkar Oriental Research Institute 64
42. Pune, Bhandarkar Oriental Research Institute 65
43. Pune, Bhandarkar Oriental Research Institute 68
44. Pune, Ānandāśrama 1546
45. Tübingen, Universitätsbibliothek I.458
46. Tübingen, Universitätsbibliothek I.459
47. Tübingen, Universitätsbibliothek I.460
48. Tübingen, Universitätsbibliothek I.474
49. Udaipur, Rajasthan Oriental Research Institute 1474
50. Varanasi, Benares Hindu University, Gaekwad Library C3688
51. Varanasi, Sarasvati Bhavan 44842
52. Varanasi, Sarasvati Bhavan Library 44870
53. Varanasi, Sarasvati Bhavan Library 108824
54. Varanasi, Sarasvati Bhavan Library 108685

References

Antonelli, Roberto 1985. "Interpretazione e critica del testo." In *L'interpretazione*, vol. 4 of *Letteratura italiana direzione di Alberto Asor Rosa*, pp. 141–243. Torino: Giulio Einaudi Editore.

Bahura, Gopal Narayan 1976. *Literary Heritage of the Rulers of Amber and Jaipur. With an Index to the Register of Manuscripts in the Pothikhana of Jaipur (I. Khasmohor Collec-*

tion). Jaipur: Maharaja Sawai Man Singh II Museum, City Palace.

Bandury, Dalia and Brahmananda Gupta (eds.) 2006. *A Descriptive Catalogue of Sanskrit Manuscripts in the Collection of the Asiatic Society, Vol. XV, Āyurvedic Manuscripts, Part I*. Calcutta: The Asiatic Society.

Banerjee, Manabendu 1987. "On Some Interesting Post-colophon Statements of Sanskrit Manuscripts Preserved in the Asiatic Society Library." In S. K. Maity and Upendra Thakur (eds.), *Indological studies: Prof. D.C. Sircar Commemoration Volume*, pp. 75–80. New Delhi: Abhinav Publications.

— 1991. "On Some Copyists of Sanskrit Manuscripts." *Journal of the Asiatic Society*, **33**, 1–14.

Bhandarkar, Ramkrishna Gopal 1884. *Report on the Search for Sanskrit Mss. in the Bombay Presidency during the years 1882–1883*. Bombay: Government Central Press.

Bühler, Curt Ferdinand 1960. *The Fifteenth-Century Book. The Scribes, the Printers, the Decorators*. Philadelphia: Univ. of Pennsylvania Press.

Bühler, Georg 1877. *Detailed Report of a Tour in Search of Sanskrit Mss. Made in Kaśmîr, Rajputana, and Central India. Extra Number of the Journal of the Bombay Branch of the Royal Asiatic Society*. Bombay and London: Society's Library and Trübner & Co.

Clemente, Michela 2007. "Colophons as Sources: Historical Information from Some Brag dkar rta so Xylographies." *Rivista di Studi Sudasiatici*, **2**, 121–58.

Colas, Gérard 1999. "The Criticism and Transmission of Texts in Classical India." *Diogenes*, **47(2)**, 30–43.

Filliozat, Jean 1941. *Catalogue du fonds sanscrit [Bibliothèque Nationale], Fasc. I*. Paris: Adrien-Maisonneuve.

Gough, Archibald Edward 1878. *Papers Relating to the Collection and Preservation of the Records of Ancient Sanskrit Literature in India*. Calcutta: Office of Superintendent of Government Printing.

Kathavate, Abaji Vishnu 1901. *Report on the Search for Sanskrit Manuscripts in the Bombay Presidency during the Years 1891/92–1894/95*. Bombay.

Meulenbeld, Gerrit Jan 1999–2002. *A History of Indian Medical Literature*, vol. XV of *Groningen Oriental Studies*. Groningen: E. Forsten. 5v.

Pasquali, Giorgio 1952. *Storia della tradizione e critica del testo*. Firenze: Felice le Monnier, 2nd edn. 1st ed. 1934.

Patel, Jashu and Krishan Kumar 2001. *Libraries and Librarianship in India*. Westport, Conn., and London: Greenwood Press.

Pingree, David E. 1997. *From Astral Omens to Astrology: from Babylon to Bīkāner*, vol. LXXVIII of *Serie Orientale Roma*. Rome: Istituto Italiano per l'Africa e l'Oriente.

Pollock, Sheldon 2001. "New Intellectuals in Seventeenth-century India." *The Indian Economic and Social History Review*, **38(1)**, 3–31.

— 2002. "Introduction: Working Papers on Sanskrit Knowledge-Systems on the Eve of Colonialism." *Journal of Indian Philosophy*, **30**, 431–39.

— 2007. "The Language of Science in Early-Modern India." In Karin Preisendanz (ed.), *Expanding and Merging Horizons. Contributions to South Asian and Cross-Cultural Studies in Commemoration of Wilhelm Halbfass*, pp. 203–20. Wien: Österreichische Akademie der Wissenschaften.

Reynolds, Leighton D. and Nigel G. Wilson 1991. *Scribes and Scholars. A Guide to the Transmission of Greek and Latin Literature*. Oxford: Clarendon Press, 3rd edn. 1st ed. 1968.

Sarma, K. V. 2001. "Manuscripts Repositories in India: An

Analytical Survey." In François Grimal (ed.), *Les sources et le temps. Sources and Time. A colloquium, Pondicherry 11–13 January 1997*, pp. 413–17. Pondicherry: Institut français de Pondichéry, École française d'Extrême-Orient.

Scherrer-Schaub, Cristina A. and George Bonani 2002. "Establishing a Typology of the Old Tibetan Manuscripts: A Multidisciplinary Approach." In Susan Whitfield (ed.), *Dunhuang Manuscript Forgeries*, pp. 184–215. London: The British Library.

Sharma, Har Dutt 1939. *Descriptive Catalogue of the Government Collections of Manuscripts deposited at the Bhandarkar Oriental Research Institute, Vol.XVI, part I, Vaidyaka*. Descriptive Catalogue of Manuscripts in the Government Manuscripts Library. Pune: Bhandarkar Oriental Research Institute.

Stark, Ulrike 2007. *An Empire of Books. The Naval Kishore Press and the Diffusion of the Printed Word in Colonial India, 1858–1895*. New Delhi: Permanent Black.

Timpanaro, Sebastiano 1975. "The Freudian Slip." *New Left Review*, **I/91**, 43–56. Translation by John Matthews. The article presents an abridged version of two chapters from: Sebastiano Timpanaro, *Il lapsus freudiano: Psicanalisi e critica testuale*. Firenze: La nuova Italia, 1974.

Vatsyayan, Kapila 2006. "Is the Unpublished Manuscript Heritage of India Relevant to Contemporary Academia?" In Sudha Gopalakrishnan (ed.), *Tattvabodha. Essays from the Lecture Series of the National Mission for Manuscripts. Vol. I*, pp. 48–56. Delhi: National Mission for Manuscripts & Munshiram Manoharlal.

2 On What to Do with a Stemma – Towards a Critical Edition of *Carakasaṃhitā Vimānasthāna* 8

Philipp A. Maas

The present paper highlights a first result of a series of research projects that aim, among other things, at a critical edition of the *Carakasaṃhitā Vimānasthāna* on the basis of more than fifty paper manuscripts from the northern part of South Asia. In taking a special focus on the application of the stemmatic method to this large textual tradition, the paper illustrates how a well-established hypothesis concerning the textual history of the *Carakasaṃhitā* is frequently useful – and in some cases even indispensable – in order to judge the genealogical relationship of different versions of

---

The present paper is a corrected, slightly revised and extended version of Maas 2009. Work on this paper has been generously supported by the Austrian Science Fund (FWF) in the context of the FWF projects P17300-G03 ("Philosophy and Medicine in Early Classical India") and P19866-G15 ("Philosophy and Medicine in Early Classical India II"). The critical edition of passages from the *Carakasaṃhitā Vimānasthāna* cited in this paper has been prepared in a close collaboration of Professor Dr Karin Preisendanz, Dr Cristina Pecchia and the present author. I would like to express my gratitude to Susanne Kammüller for having taken a close look at my English.

In what follows, the abbreviation Crit^{ed} refers to Preisendanz *et al.* in preparation, and Tri^{ed} to Ācārya 1941.

the same text. The fundamental importance of stemmatics for the editorial process may not, however, distract from the simple fact that in dealing with large and ancient traditions of Sanskrit texts the application of this method does not automatically result in the reconstruction of a historically correct textual version.

Among the sources of classical Ayurveda written in Sanskrit, the comprehensive compendium entitled *Carakasaṃhitā* figures most prominently. According to Meulenbeld's *A History of Indian Medical Literature* (1999–2002) (henceforth *HIML*), this work must have been composed between about 100 B.C. and A.D. 200.[1] The *Carakasaṃhitā* (henceforth *CS*) is very well known from a large number of printed editions, the most widely-read of which is probably the third edition by the editor Jādavji Trikamji Ācārya, published in Bombay in 1941.[2]

In 1901, forty years before Trikamji's edition appeared for the first time, the German Indologist Julius Jolly published an exposition of Indian medicine, which until today has remained one of the most reliable and comprehensive outlines of this branch of indigenous Indian science. Jolly made extensive use of the *CS* and in a somewhat casual remark he mentioned the bad state of transmission of the *CS* and the discrepancy between manuscripts and printed editions.[3] Two years later, his French colleague Palmyr Cordier remarked on the superiority of the Kashmiri recension as compared with the printed text of the vulgate.[4]

---

[1] *HIML*: 1A, 114.

[2] Ācārya 1941.

[3] Jolly 1901: 11.

[4] Cordier 1903: 329. Cordier's source was the Śāradā manuscript of the *CS* preserved at the Bhandarkar Oriental Research Institute, Pune ($P1^{ś}$). I am indebted to Karin Preisendanz for drawing my attention to Cordier's publication.

Unfortunately, these observations did not result in their natural consequence, i.e., an endeavour to prepare a critical edition of this work based on a large variety of manuscripts, presumably because of the enormous difficulties that a project aiming at a critical edition at that time would have had to cope with. At the beginning of the 20th century it was almost impossible for an individual scholar to achieve an edition based on a large variety of witnesses from different parts of the Indian subcontinent. In our time travel in South Asia has become easier and we are in the fortunate position to transform technical progress concerning the reproduction of manuscript materials and processing of large amounts of complex data into a deeper knowledge of the textual history of Sanskrit works. It was this improvement of the technical means available that made it possible, only one hundred years after the publication of the German original of Jolly's *Indian Medicine* in 1901, to initiate a series of research projects in Vienna, Austria, funded by the Austrian Science Fund, that aim at a critical edition along with an annotated English translation of the *CS*'s third book, the *Vimānasthāna*.

In the course of these projects, images of fifty-four manuscripts were collected from libraries in India, Europe and Nepal.[5] All of these manuscripts originate from the northern part of India, with the sole exception of a quite modern paper manuscript from Mysore (siglum M^k). Unfortunately, we have not yet been able to trace a single handwritten textual witness containing the *CS*'s *Vimānasthāna* in any manuscript library in South India.

With regard to scripts, the manuscripts fall into four groups: besides the aforementioned manuscript in Kannaḍa script, we have forty-three manuscripts written in

[5]See the list of "Sigla of Manuscripts" on p. 57.

Devanāgarī, nine in Bengali script and one single manuscript written in Śāradā.

In the first phase of our still-ongoing editorial work, the "collation," all textual witnesses are compared with the widely known edition of Trikamji, that we chose as our standard version. In the course of this comparison all differences in readings between the manuscripts and the text as edited by Trikamji are noted with very few exception, like, for example, *sandhi*-variants, variants of punctuation, variants of consonant gemination after "r," variants of homograph and semi-homograph *akṣaras*.

For the last couple of years, I have been working upon the final section of the *CS Vimānasthāna*, i.e., *Vi* 8.67–157 in Trikamji's edition. As a result of the work done so far, nine out of fifty-four manuscripts were found to be direct copies of other manuscripts available to us. The "Hypothetical Stemma of the *CS Vimānasthāna*" is shown in Figure 2.1.[6] Two manuscripts are in fact fragments that do not even contain the passage under investigation.

The passage *Vimānasthāna* 8.67–157 has approximately 4100 words and nominal stems in compounds. Since the collation of 52 manuscripts records ca. 4000 variants, more than 97% of all words and nominal stems in Trikamji's edition have at least one variant in one or several manuscripts. Or, to put it differently, less than three percent of Trikamji's text are transmitted without a variant in the manuscripts at our disposal. Admittedly, the majority of variants are insignificant scribal mistakes that can be corrected easily. Nev-

[6]In Fig. 2.1, continuous lines indicate direct dependence, broken lines show contamination. Sigla printed in bold type are used as group sigla for collated and critically edited text passages. This stemmatic hypothesis was superseded by the one presented in Maas 2010a: 65.

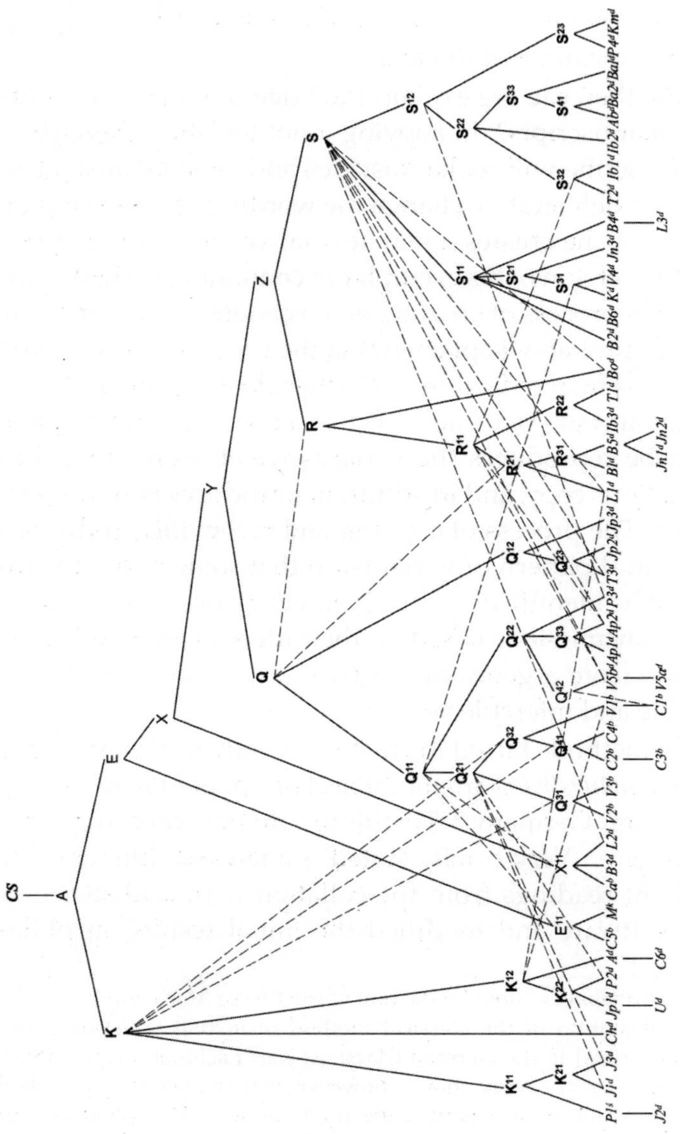

Figure 2.1: Hypothetical Stemma of the *CS Vimānasthāna* (October 2008).

ertheless, there is a considerable number of variants that affect the meaning of the text.

How then can we explain the huge number of variants in the manuscripts? In copying a not too short passage of text any scribe will make mistakes and, at some instances, may even deliberately change the wording of his exemplar. In this way, he creates a new textual version which differs from the version of his exemplar in containing variant readings. This process of creating new versions with every new copy has probably kept changing the *CS* ever since the first copy of the final redaction by Dṛḍhabala was prepared, perhaps about 1500 years ago.[7] When a new version is copied, the scribe reproduces the variants which were created in the previous copy, and in addition, introduces new variants himself. The process of copying and recopying produces a hierarchical pattern of variants, so that some variant readings can be identified as being characteristics of whole lines of the transmission. Based on their identification, it is possible to create a genealogical tree, i.e., a "stemma," of all available and inferable versions.[8]

The methods I used to create a hypothetical stemma for the *CS Vimānasthāna* are the subject of a paper I read in 2007 at Freiburg, Germany.[9] Therefore I do not want to go into details here. Very briefly stated, I analyzed different sets of variant readings from the collation with cladistic computer software and modified the initial results on philo-

---

[7] On Dṛḍhabala's "final" redaction of the *CS* see Maas 2010b: 1–4.

[8] The invention of the classical method of textual criticism is frequently ascribed to the German Classicist Karl Lachmann (1793–1851). Timpanaro (2005) clearly shows, however, that the set of rules called Lachmann's method was neither invented nor actually applied by Karl Lachmann. The theoretical principles of textual criticism have been formulated by Paul Maas (1958), Martin West (1973) and others.

[9] An extended version of this paper was published as Maas 2010a.

logical principles. The stemma presented here differs in a number of details from the stemma published in Maas 2010a, which supersedes the present one. The overall structure of both stemmata is, however, similar enough to support the following point: in critical editing it is useful to take recourse to a stemmatic hypothesis.

The development of a stemmatic hypothesis is important in all cases where external evidence for the development of a text in time does not exist, since then the evidence derived from comparing different text versions is the only source of information about the textual history of a given work. On a practical level, anyone concerned with critical editing will try to become as familiar as possible with the transmission history of the text under investigation, since this knowledge holds crucial clues for answering the often difficult question as to which version of a text is original and which version is the result of a transmissional or redactorial change. Two examples may illustrate this point.

In *Vimānasthāna* 8.96, according to Trikamji's numeration, we find a description of patients whose natural constitution (*prakṛti*) is said to be predominated by the humour (*doṣa*) phlegm. After enumerating the characteristics of phlegm, the passage continues to establish a correspondence between the essential qualities of phlegm and certain characteristics of the patient's body parts. In this context we read in all manuscripts:[10]

> *sāndratvād upacitaparipūrṇasarvagātrāḥ*
> All limbs [of the patient] are strong and full since [phlegm] is stout.

[10]Manuscripts $B5^d$ $Jn1^d$ $Jn2^d$ $Jp3^d$ do not transmit the passage under discussion due to lacunae.

Tri^{ed}	sāndratvād upacitaparipūrṇasarvāṅgāḥ
selected variants[11]	-sarvāṅgāḥ] Q^{21} Ch^d; sarvagātrāḥ K (-Ch^d) $B3^d$ $L2^d$ M^k Q^{23} Q^{22} R^{11} (-$B5^d$ $Jn1^d$ $Jn2^d$) S Bo^d; † $B5^d$ $Jn1^d$ $Jn2^d$ $Jp3^d$
Crit^{ed}	sāndratvād upacitaparipūrṇasarvagātrāḥ

Table 2.1: *CS Vi* 8.96, 6.

The manuscripts that share the inferred witness Q^{21} as their common ancestor, i.e., the Bengali manuscripts $C1^b$ $C2^b$ $C3^b$ $C4^b$ $V1^b$ $V2^b$ $V3^b$ as well as the Kashmir manuscript from Chandigarh Ch^d, read *sarvāṅgāḥ* instead of *sarvagātrāḥ* at the end of the sentence (see Table 2.1). An editor without knowledge of the transmission would have severe difficulties in deciding which of these two different readings is the original one, since they are synonyms. With a well-founded hypothesis on the transmission, however, the decision is easily made in favour of *sarvagātrāḥ*. The original was replaced by *sarvāṅgāḥ* when manuscript Q^{21} was copied, and an identical change happened in the course of the preparation of Ch^d or one of its immediate exemplars.

A stemmatic hypothesis is not only useful when decisions in favour of one out of two synonyms (or words with similar meanings) are concerned. It also allows to decide the frequently difficult question, whether a passage that is missing in one or several witnesses was part of the oldest reconstructable text.

An instructive example for this is to be found at the end of *Vimānasthāna* 8.87. This passage explains the topic *karaṇa* ("instrument") as the second out of ten topical com-

[11]For the full set of variant readings, see Appendix, p. 57 below.

plexes (*prakaraṇa*) that a physician has to examine in order to treat a patient successfully. Among the discussed "instruments," medical substances (*bheṣaja*) are said to be in need of an examination with regard to their original qualities (*guṇa*), their potency (*prabhāva*), place (*deśa*) and season (*ṛtu*) of origin, and with respect to a number of additional points, the list of which ends with the effectiveness to eliminate or to calm down the *doṣa*s. Immediately after a concluding remark, which states that besides the medical substance under investigation there are different others which could serve as an alternative, all manuscripts stemming from the inferred witness S, as well as $Ap2^d$ Bo^d $L1^d$ $T3^d$ $V5a^d$ $V5b^d$ read the following nine *anuṣṭubh*-stanzas, introduced by *bhavanti cātra*:[12]

> *ānūpaḥ prāyaśo yo 'smin deśaḥ saṃparikīrtitaḥ* |
> *ajasraṃ jāyate tatra madhuraḥ snigdhaśītalaḥ* ||1||
>
> In this respect,[13] a region known as mostly wet constantly produces an oleaginous and cool sweet flavour.
>
> *ye 'mbhaḥsamīpe deśāḥ syur nityam arkāṃśutāpitāḥ* |
> *jāyate 'mlo rasas tatra snigdhoṣṇo lavaṇas tathā* || 2 ||
>
> Regions near to water, which are permanently heated by sunlight, produce a sour and a salty flavour, which are oleaginous and hot.
>
> *alpodakāś ca ye deśā nityaṃ sūryāṃśutāpitāḥ* |
> *jāyate prāyaśas tatra rūkṣoṣṇaḥ kaṭuko rasaḥ* || 3 ||

[12] For variant readings, see Appendix, pp. 52–56.

[13] The locative pronoun *asmin* must refer to a word outside the present passage. Its occurrence here indicates that the whole passage was inserted into the *CS Vi* from a different, unidentified text.

Regions being short of water and permanently heated by sunlight, mostly produce a rough and hot sharp flavour.

asvedāś cāpi ye deśāḥ prāyeṇānilasevitāḥ |
kaṣāyatiktau tebhyo 'pi jāyete rūkṣaśītalau || 4 ||

And from regions being free from warm moisture, which frequently abound in wind, bitter and astringent flavours being rough and cool are produced.

jāyante 'nyeṣv api prāyo vyaktā deśeṣu ṣaḍ rasāḥ |
na teṣāṃ tādṛśaṃ vīryaṃ sparśo vāpy upalabhyate || 5 ||
yathā svayonau jātānāṃ mahābhūtaviśeṣataḥ |

Other regions too produce mostly the six manifest flavours, but one observes that these neither possess the same characteristic efficiency nor the same tangible quality, like beings born from their respective womb, because of specific gross elements.

santi hy anurasāḥ kecin madhurā uṣṇasaṃmatāḥ || 6 ||
yathā gokṣurako dṛṣṭaḥ svādur uṣṇaḥ svavīryataḥ |
kapittham amlam uddiṣṭaṃ tac ca rūkṣaguṇaṃ smṛtam || 7 ||

As is well known, there are some sweet secondary tastes which are regarded as hot. One sees, for example, that *Gokṣuraka* is sweet and, according to its own potency, hot. *Kapittha* is taught to be sour. And it possesses, according to the textbooks, a rough quality.

kṣāras tu lavaṇeṣv eva saṃgato rūkṣasaṃmataḥ |
sasnehāḥ sarṣapāś cāpi lakṣyante kaṭukā rase || 8 ||

> *Kṣāra* is associated with salts and is regarded as rough. And one perceives that mustard seeds, that have oil, are sharp with regard to taste.
>
> *vīśālāṃ rasataś cāhus tiktām uṣṇaguṇānvitām |*
> *uṣṇāṃ ca trivṛtām āhuḥ kaṣāyāṃ rasatas tathā* || 9 || *iti*
>
> *Vīśālā* is said to be bitter with regard to taste, and to possess a hot quality. And similarly, the hot *Trivṛt* is said to be astringent with regard to taste.

In its first four stanzas this passage describes four different regions in which special varieties of the six flavours (*rasa*) are generated: The wet region (*ānūpa*) produces an oily and cool sweet flavour, whereas hot regions, close to water produce sour and salty tastes, which are both said to be oily and hot. Dry and hot regions, on the other hand, generate a rough and hot pungent taste. Finally, windy regions "free from sweat" (*asveda*), i.e., dry and cool windy regions, are said to produce bitter and astringent flavours, which are regarded as rough and cool. Stanza 5 and 6ab state that these six tastes are also produced in other regions, but without the mentioned tangible qualities (*sparśa*) and characteristic efficiency (*vīrya*). The concluding stanzas, i.e., stanzas 6cd-9, deal with secondary tastes (*anurasa*) in a number of medical plants, which deviate in their tangible qualities and characteristic efficiency from the outline given in the first four stanzas.

The metrical passage is thematically just faintly connected with the preceding prose passage. Although it does deal with the already mentioned topics of the origin of medical substances and with their qualities as well as with their potencies, it does not refer to the topics "season of origin," "mode of collection," "preparation" etc. In terms of style, moreover, it does not fit in with the remaining discussion

Tri^{ed}	-citrakasomavalkaśatāvarī-
selected variants[13]	**-citraka-**] $L2^d$ Q R S $B3^d$; *tp.* K M^k (*see note on śatāvarī*) **-somavalka-**] $L2^d$ M^k Q R S $B3^d$ $J3^d$; K (-$J3^d$ Ch^d); *somavalkala* Ch^d **-śatāvarī-**] Q^{11} (-$Ap2^d$ $P3^d$) $B3^d$ $T2^d$ (*pc*); citraka K M^k; *om.* $L2^d$ Q^{12} R S (*ac* $T2^d$) $Ap2^d$ $P3^d$
Crit^{ed}	-somavalkacitraka-

Table 2.2: *CS Vi* 8.135, 6f.

of the ten topical complexes, which is exclusively in prose. Therefore, even without knowledge of the history of the *Vimānasthāna*'s transmission, one would suspect these nine stanzas to be of secondary origin. This suspicion can be turned – as far as possible – into certainty. Given the fact that all manuscripts stemming from the inferred witness S transmit the stanzas, one can conclude that these verses were inserted into the *CS* when S was copied. The fact that $Ap2^d$ Bo^d $L1^d$ $T3^d$ $V5b^d$ $V5a^d$ also transmit this metrical passage, must accordingly be explained as the result of horizontal transmission, i.e., contamination.

When various considerations of sense, style, and the possible course of the transmission[15] fail to provide a decisive clue in favour of one or other reading, then a stemmatic hypothesis is almost indispensable for the reconstruction of an archetypal text version. This situation occurs quite frequently within Caraka's lists of medical substances.

---

[14] For variant readings, see Appendix, p. 57.

[15] Cf. West 1973: 48.

Within a list of medical substances to be used for the preparation of emetics (*vamana*) in *CS Vimānasthāna* 8.135, Trikamji's edition lists the three substances *citraka, somavalka* and *śatāvarī* (see Table 2.2). When judging the variants of the manuscripts with recourse to the stemmatic hypothesis it becomes quite obvious that Trikamji's version differs considerably from the version of the oldest reconstructable witness, i.e., archetype A.

All manuscripts belonging to the Kashmir group as well as M^k read the two substances *citraka* and *somavalka* in inverted sequence as *somavalkacitraka*. The question, which of the two sequences is the original one, is difficult to answer. One might be tempted to conclude that the common reading of K and M^k is original, because both witnesses go back to two different hyparchetypes. In a recently published paper, I have shown, however, that substantial readings shared exclusively by M^k and K as against the rest of the transmission are the result of contamination in M^k.[16] Accordingly, no stemmatic hypothesis can provide a clue to decide whether *citrakasomavalka* or *somavalkacitraka* is the reading of archetype A.

Moreover, all manuscripts sharing the hyparchetype K as their common ancestor read *somavalkaka* or *somavalkala*, instead of *somavalka*. In this case too, the stemmatic hypothesis fails to provide any clue as to whether or not one of these readings was transmitted to K from the archetype A.[17] Nor does it provide any clue as to whether either *somavalkaka* or *somavalkala* became part of the Kashmiri ver-

[16] Maas 2010a: 90 ff.

[17] According to Maas 1958: §19, p. 18, the occurrence of an error in one out of two hyparchetypes justifies the conclusion that the archetype read the correct reading. This is not entirely correct, since Maas' conclusion does not take into consideration that the seemingly original reading may be the result of an emendation.

sion only at the time that K was copied. Nevertheless, it is quite safe to regard *somavalka* as the more original reading, simply because neither *somavalkaka* nor *somavalkala* is attested as a medical substance in standard dictionaries such as those of Monier-Williams *et al.* (1899), Böhtlingk (1879–1889), or Apte (1957–1959).

Finally, *śatāvarī* is exclusively attested by manuscripts that share the common ancestor Q^{11} either directly or as a source of contamination. It is therefore highly probable that it was the scribe of this very witness, who introduced *śatāvarī* into the list of emetic substances in *CS Vi* 8.135.

The stemmatic hypothesis is not only important to establish the correct wording of a text, it may also play an important role to detect instances, in which already the oldest reconstructible version did not contain the correct wording.

A fine example can again be found in *Vi* 8.87, in the passage mentioned above that deals with the examination of medical substances.

The version edited by Trikamji differs from the text of all manuscripts in having *puruṣasyaiva tāvantaṃ doṣam* instead of *puruṣasyaitāvantaṃ doṣam* (see Table 2.3). The latter reading is clearly preferable, since the context requires the deictic pronoun *etāvat* and not the anaphoric *tāvat*; moreover, the emphatic particle *eva* right behind *puruṣasya* is quite dispensable.

More interesting than these stylistic variants which only slightly affect the meaning of the sentence under investigation, is, however, the reading *asmin vyādhau.* Since this reading is almost exclusively attested by manuscripts that have either of the two inferred witnesses Q and R as their common ancestor,[18] it seems not to have been the reading

[18] With all likelihood, $L2^{d}$ shares the reading *vyādhāv* with Q and R because it was contaminated.

Tri[ed]	*idam evaṃprakṛtyaivaṃguṇam evaṃprabhāvam asmin deśe jātam asminn ṛtāv evaṃgṛhītam evaṃnihitam evamupaskṛtam anayā ca mātrayā yuktam asmin vyādhāv evaṃvidhasya puruṣasyaiva tāvantaṃ doṣam apakarṣaty upaśamayati vā.*
selected variants[a]	**vyādhāv**] *L2[d]* Q R; ṛtāv K (-*C6[d]* *J3[d]*) S[12] *B3[d]* *Jn3[d]*; ṛtām S[11] (-*B2[d]* *Jn3[d]*) *C6[d]*; dhā.au *C5[b]*; vyādhāv asmin ṛtau *J3[d]*; roge *M[k]*; † *B2[d]* ***puruṣasyaiva tāvantaṃ***] puruṣasyaitāvantaṃ Σ
Crit[ed]	*idam evaṃprakṛtyaivaṃguṇam evaṃprabhāvam asmin deśe jātam asminn ṛtāv evaṃgṛhītam evaṃnihitam evamupaskṛtam anayā ca mātrayā yuktam asmin vyādhāv evaṃvidhasya puruṣasyaitāvantaṃ doṣam apakarṣaty upaśamayati vā.* This [medical substance] has these qualities since it has such a nature, it has this potency, it is grown in this region and in this season, it has thus been plucked, it has thus been stored, it has thus been prepared, it is suitable in this dose, in case of this disease, for such a patient, it diminishes or pacifies a humour (*doṣa*) being of this extent.

Table 2.3: *CS Vi* 8.87, 14f.

[a]For variant readings, see Appendix, p. 50.

of the archetype A. In contrast to *asmin vyādhau*, nearly all manuscripts belonging to the Kashmir group share the variant *asminn ṛtau* "in this season." The manuscripts belonging to the S group fall into two sub-groups. All witnesses going back to the inferred manuscript S^{12} and also $Jn3^d$ agree in their reading with the Kashmir group, while the remaining witnesses of the group S^{11} read *asminn ṛtām*. The fact that *asminn ṛtāv* is transmitted along both main branches of the stemma indicates that presumably it was this reading that was transmitted in the archetype A. The reading *asminn ṛtāv* is, however, difficult to accept, since the topic "season" is dealt with right at the beginning of the passage under investigation. It is easy to conceive that the word *ṛtāv* was miscopied from its occurrence at the beginning of the passage to its present position when a scribe took a look at the wrong line of text in his exemplar. Admittedly, the initial passage deals with the medical plant's season of origin, and not with the time of the year when the medical plant is actually used. Nevertheless, would one not expect a passage dealing with the examination of medical plants to refer to disease as such, and not only to the *doṣa*s as the cause of disease?

This very problem is obviously reflected in the readings transmitted in the remaining witnesses. Manuscript $J3^d$, a Kashmiri witness strongly contaminated with a Bengali version of the *CS*, combines the two alternative variants and reads *asmin vyādhāv asminn ṛtau*. The manuscript in Kannaḍa script from Mysore (M^k) transmits *asmin roge*, instead of *asminn ṛtāv*. This variant presumably reflects a second endeavour of a scribe to correct the – in his assessment faulty – reading *ṛtāv*. Finally, the witness $C5^b$ presumably reads *dhātāv* with an illegible second consonant. *dhātau* could either be a third attempt to emend *ṛtau* or it is an erroneous reading for *vyādhau*.

Taking all our findings into consideration, we must conclude that the original version cannot be reconstructed with any certainty. *asminn ṛtāv* could be the archetypal reading, but then the investigation of medical substances in our passage would refer twice to the seasons of the year and it would not deal with diseases at all. *vyādhau*, on the other hand, was not the version of the archetype A. It is presumably a well chosen emendation, similar to the emendation *roge*. If this is true, the original version may also have contained a completely different word, which is altogether lost today.

Although in this case the stemmatic hypothesis does not provide an argument in favour of one of the variants under discussion, it proves to be helpful, since it prevents the uncritical acceptance of *asmin vyādhau* as the original reading.

The next textual passage I am going to discuss is meant to illustrate that it is by no means sufficient to determine the node of the stemma at which a variant reading may have occurred for the first time, in order to arrive at the original text. No reading may be accepted only because it is transmitted by whatever manuscripts there may be. An editor who follows a stemmatic hypothesis blindly – that is, without constant reference to the meaning of the text – is necessarily led astray.

The passage occurs within the discussion of the seventh out of the ten topical complexes (*prakaraṇa*) mentioned above, i.e., place (*deśa*), or, to be more specific, in the context of the second variety of place, viz. the diseased patient (*ātura*). For a successful medical treatment the patient has to be examined with regard to a number of specific points, among which the natural constitution (*prakṛti*) of the patient is discussed first. In this discussion appears a list of causal factors which determine the *prakṛti* of the body of an embryo. Here we read in Trikamji's edition that the "body of an embryo depends ... upon the nature of the *patient's* food and lifestyle" (see Table 2.4).

The "nature of the patient's food and lifestyle" clearly is not only an odd but a wrong reading. Which *patient* would be capable to determine the constitution of an embryo by his food and by his lifestyle?

A look at the variants in the manuscripts alone does not immediately help to solve the problem. Only nine manuscripts – $B1^{d}$ $B3^{d}$ $B5^{d}$ $C3^{b}$ $C4^{b}$ $J2^{d}$ $Jn2^{d}$ $P1^{ś}$ $P3^{d}$ – read *kālagarbhāśayaprakṛtiṃm* seemingly with two final nasal sounds, one *anusvāra* plus one labial nasal *m*. At first sight, this seems to be just a trivial scribal error, i.e., an erroneous doubling of the word final. Taking regard to the stemmatic hypothesis, one could find support for this assessment: None of the manuscripts that seem to read a double final nasal is particularly trustworthy, neither do these manuscripts form a solid genealogical group. From a purely stemmatic point of view, the double nasal would have to be judged as a case of parallelism, i.e., the independent occurrence of an identical error in different parts of the transmission. Cakrapāṇidatta's comment on this passage shows, however, that this assessment is simply wrong. His gloss *mātur āhāravihārau* "food and lifestyle of the mother" (Tri^{ed} p. 277a, l. 19) provides the decisive clue. The four mentioned manuscripts do not at all read a superfluous *anusvāra*; on the contrary, they are the only witnesses that have the original reading *mātur āhāravihāraprakṛtiṃ* "food and lifestyle of the mother" instead of *āturāhāravihāraprakṛtiṃ* "food and lifestyle of the patient," presumably because the scribes of each of them independently from the others, correctly inserted an *anusvāra* that was lost in their

Tri^{ed}	*śukraśoṇitaprakṛtiṃ kālagarbhāśayaprakṛtim* āturāhāravihāraprakṛtiṃ *mahābhūtavikāraprakṛtiṃ ca garbhaśarīram apekṣate.* The body of the embryo depends upon the nature of sperm and blood, upon the nature of time and uterus, upon the nature of the *patient's* food and lifestyle and upon the nature of the modification of the gross elements.
selected variants[a]	**kālagarbhāśayaprakṛtiṃ**] kālagarbhāśayaprakṛtiṃm *B1*^{d} *B3*^{d} *B5*^{d} *C3*^{b} *C4*^{b} *J2*^{d} *Jn2*^{d} *P1*^{ś} *P3*^{d}
Crit^{ed}	*śukraśoṇitaprakṛtiṃ kālagarbhāśayaprakṛtiṃ* mātur āhāravihāraprakṛtiṃ *mahābhūtavikāraprakṛtiṃ ca garbhaśarīram apekṣate.* The body of the embryo depends upon the nature of sperm and blood, upon the nature of time and uterus, upon the nature of the *mother's* food and lifestyle and upon the nature of the modification of the gross elements.

Table 2.4: *CS Vi* 8.95, 2–4.

[a]For variant readings, see Appendix, p. 56.

respective exemplars.[19]

I have selected the variant readings discussed so far in order to illustrate on the one hand the usefulness – and in fact the indispensability – of the application of a stemmatic hypothesis within the editorial process, and on the other hand to hint at the perils of blind trust in its results. Moreover, as we have seen, there are also cases of textual variation that escape any stemmatic analysis. Due to its very nature, even the best stemmatic hypothesis cannot provide a clue to decide which out of two hyparchetypal readings derived from the archetype. Moreover, no stemmatic hypothesis helps to reconstruct an original reading if the archetypal reading is found to be of secondary origin. And finally, numerous cases are to be met with, in which parallelism and contamination blur the picture of the transmission to such an extend that it is simply impossible to establish when and where which variant entered the transmission. But even in these cases, the editors of the *CS* are not left without help. A constant reference to the meaning of the passage under discussion, considerations of the author's (or: the authors') style, reference to parallel passages in the *CS*, in other works of Ayurveda and in Sanskrit literature in general, are the most important means for the judgement of variant readings.[20] Needless to say that their application also calls for care and caution.

---

[19]The correct reading was adopted in only two out of the more than twenty printed editions that I have examined so far, namely in those of Ācārya (1922: *Vi* 8.97, p. 315,9) (edition siglum $Bo6^E$) and Senagupta and Senagupta (1927: *Vi* 8.81, p. 1693,5) (edition siglum $C8^E$). For an online survey of printed editions of the *CS*, see `http://www.istb.univie.ac.at/caraka/Materials/120` (viewed Feb. 2011).

[20]These means are also to be applied in order to test the reliability of a hypothetical stemma.

These limitations do not, however, affect the value of the stemmatic method as such. The gain of security in the judgement of many variant readings on the basis of a well founded stemmatic hypothesis clearly justifies the enormous amount of time and energy that has to be invested in order to thoroughly collate a great number of manuscripts and to investigate their genealogical relationship in detail.

Appendix: a full collation of cited passages

NB The main text of the collation is cited from Trikamji's edition. Variant readings from the manuscripts are recorded in the apparatus, which is organized with lemmata printed in bold type. These lemmata cite the main text. Numbers in bold type refer to line numbers of the main text in prose passages. In metrical passages, the letters a, b, c and d printed in bold are used to indicate *pādas*. If lemmata refer to text occurring more than once in the same line of the main text, the lemmata are numbered consecutively. Next, all textual witnesses in support of the main text are listed, using the manuscript sigla. A semicolon separates the list of witnesses from the first variant, which in turn is followed by the sigla of witnesses that share this reading etc. Witnesses that do not transmit the variant under discussion due to a lacuna are listed at the end of each entry with a preceding dagger.

For manuscript sigla, see the listing on p. 57.

For additional signs and abbreviations, see p. 59.

CS Vi 8.87, 14f.

idaṃ evaṃprakṛtyaivaṃguṇam evaṃprabhāvam asmin deśe jātam asminn ṛtāv evaṃgṛhītam evaṃnihitam evamupaskṛtam anayā ca mātrayā yuktam asmin vyādhāv evaṃvidhasya puruṣasyaiva tāvantaṃ doṣam apakarṣaty upaśamayati vā.

87.1 idam] K (-*Jp1*^{d}) *B3*^{d} *C5*^{b} *L2*^{d} *M*^{k} Q R S (-*Km*^{d}); ivam *Km*^{d}; inavadam *Jp1*^{d} *U*^{d} **evaṃ-**[1]] K (-*A*^{d} *Pl*^{ś}) *B3*^{d} *C5*^{b} *L2*^{d} *M*^{k} Q (-*Jp2*^{d} *Jp3*^{d}) R (-*B1*^{d}) S; evaḥ *C6*^{d}; eva *A*^{d} *B1*^{d} *J2*^{d} *Jn2*^{d} *Jp3*^{d} *Pl*^{ś}; e *Jp2*^{d} **-prakṛtyaivaṃ-**] Q^{41} S (-S^{23} *V4*^{d}) *C1*^{b}; prakṛ | tyaivaṃ *V4*^{d}; prakṛtyaiva S^{23}; prakṛtyā evaṃ K (-K^{21} *Ch*^{d}) *C5*^{b} *M*^{k}; parīkṣāṃ prakṛtyā evaṃ *C6*^{d}; prakṛty evaṃ K^{21} *B3*^{d} *L2*^{d} Q^{11} (-Q^{41} *V3*^{b}) R (-*B5*^{d}); [.. .. .. ..]prakṛty evaṃ *V3*^{b}; prakṛty e[..]vaṃ *Ch*^{d}; prakṛty eva *B5*^{d} *Jn1*^{d} *Jn2*^{d}; prakṛty enaṃ Q^{23} (^{2}*pc T3*^{d}); prakṛty ena *Jp3*^{d}; ntattaty enaṃ *T3*^{d} (*ac*) **-guṇam**] K *B3*^{d} *C5*^{b} *L2*^{d} *M*^{k} Q (^{2}*pc T3*^{d}) R (-*Ib3*^{d}) S; gaṇam *Ib3*^{d}; raṇay *T3*^{d} (*ac*) **evaṃ-**[2]] K *B3*^{d} *C5*^{b} *L2*^{d} *M*^{k} Q (-*Jp2*^{d}; *pc T3*^{d}) R^{22} S (-S^{23} *B6*^{d}) *Bo*^{d}; evaṃvaṃ *Jp2*^{d}; eva S^{23} *B6*^{d}; evāṃ *T3*^{d} (*ac*); etaṃ R^{21} **-prabhāvam**] K *B3*^{d} *L2*^{d} *M*^{k} Q (-*Jp3*^{d} *T3*^{d}; *pc* *C2*^{b}) R S (-*B2*^{d} *Jn3*^{d}); prabhāv *Jn3*^{d}; prabhavam *B2*^{d} *C2*^{b} (*ac*); prābhāvam *Jp3*^{d}; .. bhāvam *C5*^{b}; - - - *T3*^{d} **asmin**] K (-*A*^{d}) *C5*^{b} *L2*^{d} *M*^{k} Q (-Q^{41}; *pc T3*^{d}) R (-*Ib3*^{d}) S; ⟨asmi⟩n *A*^{d} *C6*^{d}; asmi Q^{41} *Ib3*^{d}; asmi◊d *B3*^{d}; asmen* *T3*^{d} (*ac*) **deśe...2 asmin**] K *B3*^{d} *C5*^{b} *L2*^{d} *M*^{k} Q R (-*B5*^{d}) S; *om.* *B5*^{d} *Jn1*^{d} *Jn2*^{d} **deśe jātam asminn**] K *B3*^{d} *C5*^{b} *L2*^{d} *M*^{k} Q R (-R^{31}) S; *om.* *B1*^{d}; † *B5*^{d} *Jn1*^{d} *Jn2*^{d} **deśe**] K *B3*^{d} *L2*^{d} *M*^{k} Q (*pc C2*^{b}) R (-R^{31}) S (-*Jn3*^{d} *V4*^{d}); deśer *Jn3*^{d}; deśo *V4*^{d}; deśa *C5*^{b}; deveśe *C2*^{b} (*ac*); kṣeśe *U*^{d}; † R^{31} **jātam**] K *B3*^{d} *C5*^{b} *L2*^{d} *M*^{k} Q (-*C4*^{b}) R (-R^{31}) S; yātam *C4*^{b}; † R^{31} **asminn**] K *B3*^{d} *C5*^{b} *L2*^{d} *M*^{k} Q R (-R^{31}) S (-*Jn3*^{d}); āsmni *Jn3*^{d}; † R^{31} **ṛtāv**] K *B3*^{d} *C5*^{b} *L2*^{d} *M*^{k} Q (-*C4*^{b} *Jp3*^{d} *T3*^{d} *V5b*^{d}) S (*pc P4*^{d}) *Bo*^{d} *L1*^{d} *T1*^{d}; ṛtāṣ *P4*^{d} (*ac*); ṛtām Q^{12} (-*Jp2*^{d}) *Ib3*^{d}; ṛtov *C4*^{b}; ṛtav *V5a*^{d} *V5b*^{d}; †tān *B1*^{d}; † *B5*^{d} *Jn1*^{d} *Jn2*^{d} **2 evaṃ-**

gṛhītam] K C5^{b} L2^{d} M^{k} Q (-T3^{d}) R (-B5^{d}) S; *om.* B3^{d} T3^{d}; † B5^{d} Jn1^{d} Jn2^{d} **evaṃ-**^{1}] K C5^{b} L2^{d} M^{k} Q (-Ap1^{d} C4^{b}) R (-R^{31}) S (-B4^{d} B6^{d}); eva B1^{d} B4^{d} B6^{d} L3^{d}; avaṃ Ap1^{d} C4^{b}; *om.* B3^{d} T3^{d}; † B5^{d} Jn1^{d} Jn2^{d} **-gṛhītam**] K (-J1^{d} Jp1^{d}) C5^{b} L2^{d} M^{k} Q (-T3^{d} V3^{b} V5b^{d}) R (-B5^{d}) S (*pc* K^{d}); gṛhī-taḥm J1^{d}; gṛhītay V5b^{d}; gṛhīm Jp1^{d}; gṛhetam K^{d} (*ac*); gahītay V5a^{d}; ⟨.. ..⟩ V3^{b}; *om.* B3^{d} T3^{d}; † B5^{d} Jn1^{d} Jn2^{d} **evaṃ-**^{2}] K L2^{d} M^{k} Q (-V3^{b}) R (-B5^{d} L1^{d}) S; eva.. C5^{b}; eve B3^{d}; eva L1^{d}; *om.* V3^{b}; † B5^{d} Jn1^{d} Jn2^{d} **-nihitam**] K (-A^{d} Jp1^{d}) C5^{b} L2^{d} M^{k} Q (-Ap1^{d} C4^{b} Jp2^{d} P3^{d} V1^{b}) R (-B5^{d} L1^{d}) S^{11} (-B4^{d}); nihitam evaṃnihitam K^{12} (-P2^{d}); nihatam Jp2^{d}; vihitam B3^{d} Q^{32} (-C2^{b}) S (-S^{21} B2^{d} B6^{d}) Ap1^{d} L1^{d} P3^{d}; † B5^{d} Jn1^{d} Jn2^{d} **evam-**] K (-Ch^{d} J3^{d}) B3^{d} C5^{b} L2^{d} M^{k} Q (-C4^{b} V5b^{d}) R (-B5^{d}) S (*pc* Km^{d}); evaṃm C4^{b} Ch^{d} V5a^{d} V5b^{d}; evaṃ | m C6^{d}; evas J3^{d}; evem Km^{d} (*ac*); † B5^{d} Jn1^{d} Jn2^{d} **-upaskṛtam**] K (-Ch^{d} J1^{d}) B3^{d} C5^{b} L2^{d} M^{k} Q (-Ap1^{d} V5b^{d}) R (-R^{31}) S (-B4^{d}); upaskṛtyam J1^{d}; upaskṛ[tye]tam B4^{d}; upaskatam B1^{d} V5a^{d} V5b^{d}; upakṛtam Ap1^{d}; uraskṛtam Ch^{d}; † B5^{d} Jn1^{d} Jn2^{d} **anayā**] K (-J1^{d}) B3^{d} L2^{d} M^{k} Q (-Ap1^{d}) R (-B5^{d}) S; anayāṃ Ap1^{d}; anuyā J1^{d}; ayā C5^{b}; † B5^{d} Jn1^{d} Jn2^{d} **ca**] *om.* K B3^{d} C5^{b} L2^{d} M^{k} Q R (-B5^{d}) S; † B5^{d} Jn1^{d} Jn2^{d} **mātrayā**] K B3^{d} C5^{b} L2^{d} M^{k} Q R^{11} (-B5^{d}) S (-Km^{d}); [tra]mātrayā Bo^{d}; *om.* Km^{d}; † B5^{d} Jn1^{d} Jn2^{d} **yuktam...**Tri^{ed} 87, 18 **tac**] K B3^{d} C5^{b} L2^{d} M^{k} Q R (-B5^{d}) S (-B2^{d}); *om.* B2^{d}; † B5^{d} Jn1^{d} Jn2^{d} **yuktam**] K B3^{d} C5^{b} L2^{d} M^{k} Q (-V5b^{d}) R (-B5^{d}) S (-B2^{d}); yuktayuktam V5a^{d} V5b^{d}; † B2^{d} B5^{d} Jn1^{d} Jn2^{d} **asmin**] K (-Jp1^{d}) B3^{d} C5^{b} L2^{d} M^{k} Q R^{11} (-B5^{d}) S (-B2^{d}); asmin^{a} Bo^{d}; āsmin Jp1^{d} U^{d}; † B2^{d} B5^{d} Jn1^{d} Jn2^{d} **vyādhāv**] L2^{d} Q (-Q^{23} Ap1^{d}) R^{11}; vyādhov Bo^{d}; vyādhyāv T3^{d}; vyāyāv Jp2^{d}; cādhāṃv Ap1^{d}; ṛtāv K (-J3^{d}) B3^{d} S (-S^{31} B2^{d} B4^{d} B6^{d}); ṛtām S^{11} (-B2^{d} Jn3^{d}) C6^{d}; dhā.au C5^{b}; atām L3^{d}; vyādhāv asmin ṛtau J3^{d}; roge M^{k}; † B2^{d} **3 evaṃ-**] K (-P2^{d}) B3^{d} C5^{b} L2^{d} M^{k} Q (-V5b^{d}) R (-L1^{d}) S (-B2^{d}); eva V5a^{d} V5b^{d}; evevaṃ P2^{d}; avaṃ L1^{d}; † B2^{d} **-vidhasya**] K B3^{d} C5^{b} L2^{d} M^{k} Q R S (-B2^{d} P4^{d}); vidhaṃsya P4^{d}; † B2^{d} **puruṣasyaiva tāvantaṃ**] puruṣa-syaitāvantaṃ K C5^{b} L2^{d} M^{k} Q (-Q^{23} Ap1^{d}; *pc* C4^{b}) R (-B1^{d}) S (-B2^{d} Ib1^{d} K^{d}); puruṣasyaitāva-ttaṃ Jn2^{d}; puruṣasya etāvattaṃ B3^{d}; puruṣasyaitācataṃ Jp2^{d}; puruṣasyaitavanta B1^{d} K^{d}; puruṣasyaivantaṃ C4^{b} (*ac*); puruṣasyetāvaṃtaṃ Ap1^{d}; puruṣasyetāvattaṃ Jn1^{d}; puruṣasyai-tāmu ⁻⁻ T3^{d}; guruṣasyaitāvaṃtaṃ Ib1^{d}; † B2^{d} **doṣam**] K (-P2^{d}; *pc* Jp1^{d}) B3^{d} C5^{b} L2^{d} M^{k} Q (-Q^{41} Ap1^{d} T3^{d}) R S (-B2^{d}); dośaṃm Q^{41} Ap1^{d}; dauṣam K^{22} (*ac* Jp1^{d}); ⁻ ⁻ m T3^{d}; † B2^{d} **apa-**] K B3^{d} C5^{b} L2^{d} M^{k} Q (-T3^{d}) R (-R^{31}; *pc* Jn2^{d}) S^{21} B6^{d} Ib2^{d}; a B4^{d} L3^{d}; upa S^{12} (-Ib2^{d}) B5^{d} Jn2^{d} (*ac*) T3^{d}; ana B1^{d}; † B2^{d} **-karṣaty**] C5^{b} S (-B2^{d}) Ib3^{d}; karṣayaty K B3^{d} L2^{d} M^{k} Q (-Ap1^{d} C2^{b}) R (-B1^{d} Ib3^{d}); karṣayaṃty Ap1^{d}; karṣany L3^{d}; karṣa C2^{b} C3^{b}; rthayam B1^{d}; † B2^{d} **upa-**] K B3^{d} C5^{b} L2^{d} M^{k} Q R (-Ib3^{d}) S (-B2^{d}); apa Ib3^{d}; † B2^{d} **-śamayati**] K B3^{d} C5^{b} L2^{d} M^{k} Q^{11} (-Q^{32}) S (-Ab^{d} B2^{d} P4^{d}) Bo^{d} Jp3^{d} T1^{d} (^{2}*pc*); śamayasi Ab^{d}; śamamṃyāti Q^{32} (-C2^{b}); śamaṃ-mati C2^{b} C3^{b}; śayati B1^{d}; śemayati P4^{d}; śaya iti Jn1^{d} L1^{d}; śama iti Jn2^{d}; samayati Q^{23}; sama-bhati B5^{d}; rūpayati R^{22} (*ac* T1^{d}); † B2^{d} **vā**] K C5^{b} M^{k} Q^{21}; cā B3^{d} B6^{d} Ba2^{d} Ib1^{d} Ib2^{d} Jn3^{d}; ca L2^{d} Q^{22} S (-B2^{d} B6^{d} Ba2^{d} Ib1^{d} Ib2^{d} Jn3^{d} Km^{d}) T1^{d}; *om.* Q^{12} R (-T1^{d}) Km^{d}; † B2^{d}

Interpolated passage after 8.87,19 in *S Ap2^d Bo^d L1^d T1^d (^2pc) T3^d V5a^d V5b^d* [21]

bhavanti cātra —

> ānūpaḥ prāyaśo yo 'smin deśaḥ saṃparikīrtitaḥ |
> ajasraṃ jāyate tatra madhuraḥ snigdhaśītalaḥ ‖ 1 ‖

1 **cātra**] S (-$B6^d$; ^2pc Ab^d) $Ap2^d$ Bo^d $L1^d$ $T1^d$ (^2pc) $T3^d$ $V5a^d$ $V5b^d$; cāca Ab^d (*ac*); cātra ślokāḥ $B6^d$ **a ānūpaḥ**] S (-S^{23}) $Ap2^d$ Bo^d $L1^d$ $T1^d$ (^2pc) $V5a^d$ $V5b^d$; ānūpa S^{23}; ānuprā $T3^d$ **prāyaśo**] S (-$B2^d$) $Ap2^d$ Bo^d $L1^d$ $T1^d$ (^2pc); prāyaṃśo $L3^d$; prāyaso $B2^d$ $V5a^d$ $V5b^d$; paśe ⁻ $T3^d$ **yo 'smin**] S (-S^{31} $B2^d$ $B6^d$ $P4^d$) $Ap2^d$ $L1^d$ $T1^d$ (^2pc); yosmi $B6^d$; yāsmin K^d; ye yo smin $P4^d$; yasmin $B2^d$ Bo^d $V4^d$; so 'smin* $V5a^d$ $V5b^d$; ⁻ ⁻ ⁻ $T3^d$ **b deśaḥ**] S (-K^d) $Ap2^d$ Bo^d $L1^d$ $T1^d$ (^2pc) $V5a^d$ $V5b^d$; deśa K^d; daśaḥ $T3^d$ **saṃparikīrtitaḥ**] $Ap2^d$; sa parikīrtitaḥ S (-K^d) Bo^d $L1^d$ $T1^d$ (^2pc) $V5b^d$; sa parikartitaḥ $V5a^d$; .m aparikīrtitaḥ K^d; parīkirttitaḥ $T3^d$ **c ajasraṃ**] S (-$Ba2^d$ $Ib1^d$) $Ap2^d$ Bo^d $L1^d$ $T1^d$ (^2pc); ajasra $T3^d$; ajasvaṃ $Ba2^d$; ajastvaṃ $Ib1^d$; bhajasraṃ $V5a^d$ $V5b^d$ **jāyate**] S $Ap2^d$ Bo^d $L1^d$ $T1^d$ (^2pc) $T3^d$; jāyeta $V5a^d$ $V5b^d$ **tatra**] S (-$Ba2^d$) $Ap2^d$ Bo^d $L1^d$ $T1^d$ (^2pc) $T3^d$ $V5a^d$ $V5b^d$; tra $Ba2^d$ **d madhuraḥ**] S^{11} (-S^{31}) $Ap2^d$ Bo^d $T3^d$ $V5a^d$ $V5b^d$; madhuraṃ $Ib2^d$; madhura S (-$B2^d$ $B4^d$ $B6^d$ $Ib2^d$ $Jn3^d$) $L1^d$ $T1^d$ (^2pc) **snigdha-**] S (-$V4^d$) $Ap2^d$ Bo^d $L1^d$ $T1^d$ (^2pc) $T3^d$ $V5b^d$; snigdhaṃ $V4^d$; snidha $V5a^d$ **-śītalaḥ**] S (-$Ib2^d$) $Ap2^d$ Bo^d $L1^d$ $T1^d$ (^2pc) $T3^d$ $V5a^d$ $V5b^d$; śītalaṃ $Ib2^d$

> ye 'mbhaḥsamīpe deśāḥ syur nityam arkāṃśutāpitāḥ |
> jāyate 'mlo rasas tatra snigdhoṣṇo lavaṇas tathā ‖ 2 ‖

a **ye**] S $Ap2^d$ $L1^d$ $T1^d$ (^2pc) $V5a^d$ $V5b^d$; ya $T3^d$; yo Bo^d **'mbhaḥ-**] S (-$Ib1^d$ K^d) $Ap2^d$ $L1^d$ $T1^d$ (^2pc) $T3^d$ $V5b^d$; ṃ[tta]⟨bha⟩de Bo^d; bhaḥ $Ib1^d$ K^d $V5a^d$ **-samīpe**] S (-S^{23}) $Ap2^d$ $T1^d$ (^2pc) $T3^d$ $V5a^d$ $V5b^d$; samīpa S^{23}; samipe Bo^d; saṃmīpe $L1^d$ **deśāḥ syur**] $Ap2^d$ $B2^d$ $B6^d$ $P4^d$ $T1^d$ (^2pc); deśāḥ syu $Ib2^d$; deśā syur Ab^d Km^d $T3^d$ $V5a^d$ $V5b^d$; deśā syuḥr $L1^d$; deśā syu S (-S^{23} Ab^d $B2^d$ $B6^d$ $Ib2^d$); deśe Bo^d **b arkāṃśu-**] S (-Km^d $V4^d$) $Ap2^d$ Bo^d $L1^d$ $T1^d$ (^2pc) $T3^d$; arkāśu Km^d; athāṃśu $V4^d$; ekāṃśu $V5a^d$ $V5b^d$ **-tāpitāḥ…3b.1 sūryāṃśu-**] S $Ap2^d$ (*pc*) Bo^d $L1^d$ $T1^d$ (^2pc) $T3^d$ $V5a^d$ $V5b^d$; *om.* $Ap2^d$ (*ac*) **-tāpitāḥ**] S (-$B2^d$) $Ap2^d$ (*pc*) Bo^d $L1^d$ $T1^d$ (^2pc) $T3^d$; tāpitā $B2^d$; tāpritāḥ $V5a^d$ $V5b^d$; † $Ap2^d$ (*ac*) **c jāyate**] S (-S^{33} S^{32} $B4^d$) Bo^d $L1^d$ $T1^d$ (^2pc) $T3^d$ $V5a^d$ $V5b^d$; jāyaṃte S^{22} (-$Ib2^d$) $Ap2^d$ (*pc*) $B4^d$ $L3^d$; † $Ap2^d$ (*ac*) **'mlo**] S (-K^d) $Ap2^d$ (*pc*) Bo^d $L1^d$ $T1^d$ (^2pc) $T3^d$ (*pc*) $V5a^d$ $V5b^d$; ślo K^d; allo $T3^d$ (*ac*); † $Ap2^d$ (*ac*) **tatra**] S (-Ab^d $B2^d$) $Ap2^d$ (*pc*) Bo^d $L1^d$ $T1^d$ (^2pc) $T3^d$ $V5a^d$ $V5b^d$; ta[ra]tra Ab^d; tastūva $B2^d$; † $Ap2^d$ (*ac*) **d snigdhoṣṇo**] *em.*; snigdhoṣṇa S (-$Ib2^d$) $Ap2^d$ (*pc*) Bo^d $T1^d$ (^2pc); snidhoṣṇa $V5a^d$; snidhoṣṭhyā $V5b^d$; snigdhoha $L1^d$; snigdhe ⁻ ⁻ $T3^d$; sa snigdho $Ib2^d$; † $Ap2^d$ (*ac*) **lavaṇas**] S (*pc* $V4^d$) $Ap2^d$ (*pc*) Bo^d $L1^d$ $T1^d$ (^2pc) $T3^d$; lavaṇos $V4^d$ (*ac*); lavarās $V5a^d$ $V5b^d$; vaṇas $L3^d$; † $Ap2^d$ (*ac*)

---

[21] Stanzas are not numbered in the manuscripts.

alpodakāś ca ye deśā nityaṃ sūryāṃśutāpitāḥ |
jāyate prāyaśas tatra rūkṣoṣṇaḥ kaṭuko rasaḥ ‖ 3 ‖

a **alpodakāś**] S (-*Ba1*^{d} *V4*^{d}) *Ap2*^{d} (*pc*) *Bo*^{d} *L1*^{d} *T1*^{d} (^{2}*pc*) *T3*^{d}; [..]alpodakāś *V4*^{d}; alpodakaś *V5a*^{d} *V5b*^{d}; śnalpodakāś *Ba1*^{d}; † *Ap2*^{d} (*ac*) **ca**] S *Ap2*^{d} (*pc*) *Bo*^{d} *L1*^{d} *T1*^{d} (^{2}*pc*) *T3*^{d}; caś ca *V5b*^{d}; caś ya *V5a*^{d}; † *Ap2*^{d} (*ac*) **ye**] S (-*Ba2*^{d}) *Ap2*^{d} (*pc*) *Bo*^{d} *L1*^{d} *T1*^{d} (^{2}*pc*) *T3*^{d}; yo *V5a*^{d} *V5b*^{d}; *om.* *Ba2*^{d}; † *Ap2*^{d} (*ac*) **deśā…4a.1 ye**] S^{11} (-*B4*^{d}) S^{32} *Ap2*^{d} *Bo*^{d} *L1*^{d} *T1*^{d} (^{2}*pc*) *T3*^{d} *V5a*^{d} *V5b*^{d}; *om.* S (-S^{21} S^{32} *B2*^{d} *B6*^{d}) **deśā**] *Ap2*^{d} (*pc*) *B2*^{d} *B6*^{d} *Bo*^{d} *Jn3*^{d} *L1*^{d} *T1*^{d} (^{2}*pc*) *T2*^{d} *T3*^{d}; deśāḥ *Ib1*^{d} *V4*^{d}; deśo *K*^{d}; deśa† *V5a*^{d} *V5b*^{d}; † S (-S^{21} S^{32} *B2*^{d} *B6*^{d}) *Ap2*^{d} (*ac*) **b** **nityaṃ…3c.1 jāyate**] S^{11} (-*B4*^{d}) S^{32} *Ap2*^{d} (*pc*) *Bo*^{d} *L1*^{d} *T1*^{d} (^{2}*pc*) *T3*^{d}; *om.* *V5a*^{d} *V5b*^{d}; † S (-S^{21} S^{32} *B2*^{d} *B6*^{d}) *Ap2*^{d} (*ac*) **nityaṃ**] S^{11} (-*B4*^{d}) S^{32} *Ap2*^{d} (*pc*) *L1*^{d} *T3*^{d}; nitya *Bo*^{d} *T1*^{d} (^{2}*pc*); † S (-S^{21} S^{32} *B2*^{d} *B6*^{d}) *Ap2*^{d} (*ac*) *V5a*^{d} *V5b*^{d} **sūryāṃśu-**] S^{21} S^{32} *Ap2*^{d} (*pc*) *B6*^{d} *Bo*^{d} *L1*^{d} *T1*^{d} (^{2}*pc*) *T3*^{d}; sūryāṃsu *B2*^{d}; † S (-S^{21} S^{32} *B2*^{d} *B6*^{d}) *Ap2*^{d} (*ac*) *V5a*^{d} *V5b*^{d} **-tāpitāḥ**] S^{11} (-*B4*^{d} *V4*^{d}) S^{32} *Ap2*^{d} *Bo*^{d} *L1*^{d} *T1*^{d} (^{2}*pc*) *T3*^{d}; tāṃpitāḥ *V4*^{d}; † S (-S^{21} S^{32} *B2*^{d} *B6*^{d}) *V5a*^{d} *V5b*^{d} **c** **jāyate**] S^{11} (-*B4*^{d} *V4*^{d}) *Ap2*^{d} *Bo*^{d} *T3*^{d}; [..]jāyate *V4*^{d}; jāyaṃte S^{32} *L1*^{d} *T1*^{d} (^{2}*pc*); † S (-S^{21} S^{32} *B2*^{d} *B6*^{d}) *V5a*^{d} *V5b*^{d} **prāyaśas**] S^{21} S^{32} *Ap2*^{d} *B6*^{d} *Bo*^{d} *L1*^{d} *T1*^{d} (^{2}*pc*); prāyaśaḥs *T3*^{d}; prāyastas *B2*^{d}; †śas *V5a*^{d} *V5b*^{d}; † S (-S^{21} S^{32} *B2*^{d} *B6*^{d}) **d** **rūkṣoṣṇaḥ**] *Bo*^{d}; rūkṣoṣṇa S^{11} (-*B4*^{d}) S^{32} *Ap2*^{d} *L1*^{d} *T1*^{d} (^{2}*pc*) *T3*^{d} *V5a*^{d} *V5b*^{d}; † S (-S^{21} S^{32} *B2*^{d} *B6*^{d}) **kaṭuko**] S^{11} (-*B4*^{d}) *Ap2*^{d} *Bo*^{d} *T3*^{d} *V5a*^{d} *V5b*^{d}; kaṭukā S^{32} *L1*^{d} *T1*^{d} (^{2}*pc*); † S (-S^{21} S^{32} *B2*^{d} *B6*^{d}) **rasaḥ**] S^{11} (-*B4*^{d}) *Ap2*^{d} *Bo*^{d} *T3*^{d} *V5a*^{d} *V5b*^{d}; rasāḥ S^{32} *L1*^{d} *T1*^{d} (^{2}*pc*); † S (-S^{21} S^{32} *B2*^{d} *B6*^{d})

asvedāś cāpi ye deśāḥ prāyeṇānilasevitāḥ |
kaṣāyatiktau tebhyo 'pi jāyete rūkṣaśītalau ‖ 4 ‖

a **asvedāś**] *B2*^{d} *B6*^{d} *L1*^{d}; asvedā S^{32}; aśvedāś S^{21} *Ap2*^{d} *T1*^{d} (^{2}*pc*) *T3*^{d} *V5a*^{d} *V5b*^{d}; āsvedāś *Bo*^{d}; † S (-S^{21} S^{32} *B2*^{d} *B6*^{d}) **ye**] S^{11} (-*B4*^{d}) S^{32} *Ap2*^{d} *Bo*^{d} *L1*^{d} *T1*^{d} (^{2}*pc*) *V5a*^{d} *V5b*^{d}; *om.* *T3*^{d}; † S (-S^{21} S^{32} *B2*^{d} *B6*^{d}) **deśāḥ**] S (-S^{31} *B4*^{d} *B6*^{d}) *Ap2*^{d} *T3*^{d}; deśā S^{11} (-*B2*^{d} *Jn3*^{d}; *pc* *B4*^{d}) *Bo*^{d} *L1*^{d} *T1*^{d} (^{2}*pc*) *V5a*^{d} *V5b*^{d}; doṣā *B4*^{d} (*ac*) **b** **prāyeṇānila-**] S *Ap2*^{d} *Bo*^{d} *L1*^{d} *T1*^{d} (^{2}*pc*); proyeṇani† *V5a*^{d} *V5b*^{d}; prāyeṇ.‐‐‐ *T3*^{d} **-sevitāḥ…5c.1 tādṛśaṃ**] S *Ap2*^{d} *Bo*^{d} *L1*^{d} *T1*^{d} (^{2}*pc*) *T3*^{d}; *om.* *V5a*^{d} *V5b*^{d} **-sevitāḥ**] S (-*Km*^{d} *V4*^{d}) *Ap2*^{d} *Bo*^{d} *L1*^{d} *T1*^{d} (^{2}*pc*) *T3*^{d}; [(k).])sevitāḥ *V4*^{d}; semvitāḥ *Km*^{d}; † *V5a*^{d} *V5b*^{d} **c** **-tiktau**] S (-*Ib1*^{d}) *Ap2*^{d} *Bo*^{d} *L1*^{d} *T1*^{d} (^{2}*pc*); tiktau [|] *T3*^{d}; tikto *Ib1*^{d}; † *V5a*^{d} *V5b*^{d} **tebhyo 'pi**] S (-*Ba1*^{d}) *Ap2*^{d} *Bo*^{d} *L1*^{d} *T1*^{d} (^{2}*pc*) *T3*^{d}; tabhyo pi *Ba1*^{d}; † *V5a*^{d} *V5b*^{d} **d** **jāyete…7d.1 -guṇaṃ**] S *Ap2*^{d} *Bo*^{d} *L1*^{d} *T1*^{d} (^{2}*pc*); *rp.* *T3*^{d} (*cf. note on* smṛtam *in* 7d *below*); † *V5a*^{d} *V5b*^{d} **jāyete**] S (-S^{31} *B4*^{d} *B6*^{d}) *Ap2*^{d} *T1*^{d} (^{2}*pc*); jāyate S^{11} (-*B2*^{d} *Jn3*^{d}) *Bo*^{d} *L1*^{d} *T3*^{d}; yate *T3*^{d} (*vl*); † *V5a*^{d} *V5b*^{d} **rūkṣa-**] S (-*B4*^{d}) *Ap2*^{d} *Bo*^{d} *L1*^{d} *T1*^{d} (^{2}*pc*) *T3*^{d}; rukṣa *B4*^{d} *L3*^{d}; † *V5a*^{d} *V5b*^{d} **-śītalau**] S (-*K*^{d}) *Ap2*^{d} *Bo*^{d} *L1*^{d} *T1*^{d} (^{2}*pc*) *T3*^{d}; śītalyau *K*^{d}; śītalau | jāyaṃte rūkṣaśīta *T3*^{d} (*vl*); † *V5a*^{d} *V5b*^{d}

jāyante 'nyeṣv api prāyo vyaktā deśeṣu ṣaḍ rasāḥ |
na teṣāṃ tādṛśaṃ vīryaṃ sparśo vāpy upalabhyate ‖ 5 ‖

a **jāyante**] S (-S^{23} $B4^d$ $Ba1^d$ $Ba2^d$) $Ap2^d$ $L1^d$ $T1^d$ (^{2}*pc*) $T3^d$ (*vl*); jāyate S^{33} (-Ab^d) S^{23} $B4^d$ Bo^d $L3^d$; jā[yāṃ]〈yaṃ〉te $T3^d$; † $V5a^d$ $V5b^d$ **'nyeṣv**] S (-S^{23} S^{31}) $Ap2^d$ Bo^d $L1^d$ $T1^d$ (^{2}*pc*); nyeṣ S^{23}; 'nye py $T3^d$; ṣv S^{31}; *om.* $T3^d$ (*vl*); † $V5a^d$ $V5b^d$ **api**] S $Ap2^d$ $L1^d$ $T1^d$ (^{2}*pc*) $T3^d$; abhi Bo^d; † $V5a^d$ $V5b^d$ **b** **vyaktā**] S (-$B2^d$) $Ap2^d$ Bo^d; vyakta $B2^d$ $L1^d$ $T1^d$ (^{2}*pc*); vyukkā $T3^d$ (*vl*); pyuktā $T3^d$; † $V5a^d$ $V5b^d$ **ṣaḍ**] S Bo^d $L1^d$ $T1^d$ (^{2}*pc*) $T3^d$; yad $Ap2^d$; ḍ $L3^d$; † $V5a^d$ $V5b^d$ **rasāḥ**] S (-K^d Km^d) $Ap2^d$ Bo^d $L1^d$ $T1^d$ (^{2}*pc*) $T3^d$ (*vl*); ravasā $T3^d$; [kā]sāḥ Km^d; usāḥ K^d; † $V5a^d$ $V5b^d$ **c** **tādṛśaṃ**] S (-$Ib1^d$ Km^d; *pc* $P4^d$) $Ap2^d$ $T3^d$; tādṛśa Km^d; tādṛṣāṃ $P4^d$ (*ac*); tādāsaṃ $L3^d$; tāvṛśaṃ $T3^d$ (*vl*); vādṛśaṃ Bo^d; dṛśaṃ $Ib1^d$; dṛśyate $L1^d$ $T1^d$ (^{2}*pc*); † $V5a^d$ $V5b^d$ **vīryaṃ**] S $Ap2^d$ $L1^d$ $T1^d$ (^{2}*pc*) $T3^d$; vīrya $T3^d$ (*vl*); vīryāṃ Bo^d; †ryaṃ $V5b^d$; †rya $V5a^d$ **d** **sparśo**] S (-$B6^d$ $T2^d$) $Ap2^d$ Bo^d $T1^d$ (^{2}*pc*) $T3^d$ $V5a^d$ $V5b^d$; sparśā $B6^d$; śpaso $T2^d$; tyarśo $L1^d$ **vāpy…7a.1 yathā**] S $Ap2^d$ Bo^d $L1^d$ $T1^d$ (^{2}*pc*) $T3^d$; *rp.* $V5a^d$ $V5b^d$ (*cf. note on* gokṣurako *in* 7a *below*) **vāpy**] S $Ap2^d$ Bo^d $L1^d$ $T1^d$ (^{2}*pc*) $T3^d$ $V5b^d$; cāpy $V5a^d$ $V5b^d$ (*vl*); yāpy $T3^d$ (*vl*) **upalabhyate**] S $Ap2^d$ Bo^d $L1^d$ $T1^d$ (^{2}*pc*); upalaḥ - - $T3^d$; upakalate $V5b^d$; upakalate te $V5a^d$ $V5b^d$ (*vl*)

yathā svayonau jātānāṃ mahābhūtaviśeṣataḥ |
santi hy anurasāḥ kecin madhurā uṣṇasaṃmatāḥ ‖ 6 ‖

a **yathā**] S $Ap2^d$ Bo^d $L1^d$ $T1^d$ (^{2}*pc*) $T3^d$ (*vl*) $V5a^d$ $V5b^d$; - thā $T3^d$ **svayonau**] S $Ap2^d$ Bo^d $T1^d$ (^{2}*pc*); svayono $V5a^d$ $V5b^d$; smayottau $L1^d$; stathaunau $T3^d$; - - - $T3^d$ (*vl*) **jātānāṃ**] S (-$B6^d$ $Ba2^d$ K^d) $Ap2^d$ Bo^d $L1^d$ $T1^d$ (^{2}*pc*) $T3^d$ $V5a^d$ $V5b^d$; jā[ṃ]tānāṃ $B6^d$; jātāyāṃ $Ba2^d$; jāsānāṃ K^d **b** **mahābhūta-**] S $Ap2^d$ Bo^d $L1^d$ $T1^d$ (^{2}*pc*) $T3^d$ $V5a^d$ $V5b^d$ (*vl*); mahabhūta $V5b^d$ **c** **santi**] S $Ap2^d$ $L1^d$ $T1^d$ (^{2}*pc*) $T3^d$ $V5b^d$; samati Bo^d; ṣati $V5a^d$ $V5b^d$ (*vl*) **hy**] S $Ap2^d$ Bo^d $L1^d$ $T1^d$ (^{2}*pc*) $T3^d$ $V5b^d$; s $V5a^d$ **anurasāḥ**] S^{12} (-Km^d) $Ap2^d$ Bo^d (*pc*) $L1^d$ $T3^d$ (*vl*) $V5b^d$; anurasā S (-S^{22} $P4^d$) Bo^d (*ac*) $T1^d$ (^{2}*pc*); avurasāḥ $V5a^d$ $V5b^d$ (*vl*); atvarasā $T3^d$ **kecin**] S $Ap2^d$ Bo^d $L1^d$ $T1^d$ (^{2}*pc*) $V5a^d$ $V5b^d$; keci $T3^d$ (*vl*); kevi $T3^d$ **d** **madhurā**] S (-$Ib1^d$) $Ap2^d$ Bo^d $L1^d$ $T1^d$ (^{2}*pc*); madhu $V5a^d$ $V5b^d$; madurān $T3^d$; madurāt $T3^d$ (*vl*); pradhurā $Ib1^d$ **uṣṇa-**] S $Ap2^d$ Bo^d $L1^d$ $T1^d$ (^{2}*pc*); uṣṭḥa $V5b^d$; uṣu $T3^d$; ukṣaṣṇa $V5a^d$ $V5b^d$ (*vl*) **-saṃmatāḥ**] S (-S^{33} $Ib2^d$) $Ap2^d$ $T1^d$ (^{2}*pc*) $T3^d$ $V5a^d$ $V5b^d$; saṃmataraḥ $L1^d$; saṃgatāḥ Bo^d $Ib2^d$; saṃbhṛtāḥ Ab^d; saṃbhatāḥ S^{33} (-Ab^d)

yathā gokṣurako dṛṣṭaḥ svādur *uṣṇaḥ sva*vīryataḥ |
kapittham amlam uddiṣṭaṃ tac ca rūkṣaguṇaṃ smṛtam || 7 ||

a **gokṣurako**] S $Ap2^d$ Bo^d $L1^d$ $T1^d$ (^{2}*pc*) $T3^d$; go cāpy…yathā gokṣurako $V5a^d$ $V5b^d$ (*cf. rp. in note on* vāpy…yathā *in* 5d *above*) **dṛṣṭaḥ**] S $Ap2^d$ Bo^d $T3^d$ $V5a^d$ $V5b^d$; [dṛṣyaḥ]⟨dṛṣṭaḥ⟩ $T1^d$ (^{2}*pc*); dṛṣṭā $T3^d$ (*vl*); vṛṣya $L1^d$ **b** **svādur**] S (-Km^d; *pc* $Ib2^d$) $Ap2^d$ Bo^d $L1^d$ $T1^d$ (^{2}*pc*) $T3^d$ $V5a^d$ $V5b^d$; savur Km^d; svārud $Ib2^d$ (*ac*) **uṣṇaḥ sva-**] $B2^d$ $B6^d$ Bo^d; *uṣṇaś ca* S^{12} (-Km^d) $Ap2^d$ $T1^d$ (^{2}*pc*) $V5a^d$ $V5b^d$; uṣṇaścī Km^d; uṣṇasva $B4^d$ $Jn3^d$ $L1^d$ $L3^d$; uṣṇasya $V4^d$; ūṣṇasya K^d; uṣṇasta $T3^d$ (*vl*); uṣṇatra $T3^d$ **-vīryataḥ**] S $Ap2^d$ $L1^d$ $T1^d$ (^{2}*pc*) $T3^d$ $V5a^d$ $V5b^d$; vīryatā $T3^d$ (*vl*); vīryajaḥ Bo^d **c** **kapittham**] S $Ap2^d$ Bo^d $L1^d$ $T1^d$ (^{2}*pc*) $V5a^d$ $V5b^d$; kapitham $T3^d$ (*vl*); kadi[stha]⟨tya⟩m $T3^d$ **amlam**] S (-K^d) $Ap2^d$ Bo^d $L1^d$ $T1^d$ (^{2}*pc*) $T3^d$ $V5b^d$; amla K^d $T3^d$ (*vl*); a..m $V5a^d$ **uddiṣṭaṃ**] S (-$T2^d$) $Ap2^d$ Bo^d $L1^d$ $T1^d$ (^{2}*pc*) $V5a^d$ $V5b^d$; uddiṣṭaḥ $T2^d$; tu diṣṭaṃ $T3^d$ (*vl*); u ˉ ˉ $T3^d$ **d** **tac ca**] S $Ap2^d$ Bo^d $L1^d$ $V5a^d$ $V5b^d$; tatra $T1^d$ (^{2}*pc*); tadya $T3^d$ (*vl*); ˉ ˉ $T3^d$ **rūkṣa-**] S (-Ab^d $B4^d$ Km^d) $Ap2^d$ $T1^d$ (^{2}*pc*) $T3^d$ $V5a^d$ $V5b^d$; rūkṣ*ṇa Bo^d; rukṣa Ab^d $B4^d$ $L1^d$ $L3^d$ $T3^d$ (*vl*); nūkṣa Km^d **-guṇaṃ**] S (-$Ib1^d$) $Ap2^d$ Bo^d $L1^d$ $T1^d$ (^{2}*pc*) $V5a^d$ $V5b^d$; guṇa $Ib1^d$ $T3^d$; gu ˉ $T3^d$ (*vl*) **smṛtam**] S (-Km^d) $Ap2^d$ Bo^d $L1^d$ $T1^d$ (^{2}*pc*) $V5a^d$ $V5b^d$; smṛta Km^d; smṛtaṃ || yate…gu ˉ ˉ ˉ $T3^d$ (*cf. rp. in note on* jāyete…guṇaṃ *in* 4d *above*)

kṣāras tu lavaṇeṣv eva saṃgato rūkṣasaṃmataḥ |
sasnehāḥ sarṣapāś cāpi lakṣyante kaṭukā rase || 8 ||

a **kṣāras…9d.1 tathā**] S $Ap2^d$ Bo^d $L1^d$ $T1^d$ (^{2}*pc*) $V5a^d$ $V5b^d$; *tp.* $T3^d$ (*to* mohayitum *in* Vimānasthāna 8.82,3) **lavaṇeṣv eva**] S (-$Ba2^d$ $Ib2^d$ $P4^d$) $Ap2^d$ Bo^d $L1^d$ $T1^d$ (^{2}*pc*) $V5b^d$; lavaṇoṣeva $P4^d$; lavaṇeṣ $V5a^d$; lavaṇetheva $Ba2^d$ $T3^d$; kṣāras tu $Ib2^d$ **b** **saṃgato**] S (-$P4^d$) $Ap2^d$ Bo^d $T1^d$ (^{2}*pc*) $T3^d$ $V5a^d$ $V5b^d$; saṃgāto $L1^d$; ˉ gaṃto $P4^d$ **rūkṣa-**] S (-$B4^d$ $Ba2^d$) $Ap2^d$ Bo^d $T1^d$ (^{2}*pc*) $T3^d$; rūkṣma $V5b^d$; rukṣa $B4^d$ $Ba2^d$ $L1^d$ $L3^d$; rukṣma $V5a^d$ **-saṃmataḥ**] S $Ap2^d$ Bo^d $T1^d$ (^{2}*pc*) $V5a^d$ $V5b^d$; saṃnmataḥ $T3^d$; saṃsmṛtaḥ $L1^d$ **c** **sasnehāḥ**] S (-S^{23} S^{31}) $Ap2^d$ Bo^d $L1^d$ $T1^d$ (^{2}*pc*) $T3^d$; sasnehā S^{31}; rusnohāḥ Km^d; rusnehāḥ $P4^d$; snehāḥ $V5a^d$ $V5b^d$ **sarṣapāś**] S $Ap2^d$ Bo^d $L1^d$ $T1^d$ (^{2}*pc*); sarṣapaś $T3^d$; sasarvaṣāyāś $V5a^d$ $V5b^d$ **cāpi**] S $Ap2^d$ Bo^d $L1^d$ $T1^d$ (^{2}*pc*) $T3^d$; rāyi $V5a^d$ $V5b^d$ **d** **lakṣyante**] S (-$B2^d$) $Ap2^d$ $L1^d$ $T1^d$ (^{2}*pc*); lakṣyaṃ $T3^d$; lakṣante $B2^d$ $V5a^d$ $V5b^d$; lavaṇaṃ te Bo^d **kaṭukā**] S (-$P4^d$) $Ap2^d$ Bo^d $L1^d$ $T1^d$ (^{2}*pc*) $T3^d$ $V5a^d$ $V5b^d$; kuṃṭurukā $P4^d$ **rase**] S $Ap2^d$ Bo^d $L1^d$ $T1^d$ (^{2}*pc*) $T3^d$ (*pc*) $V5a^d$ $V5b^d$; raso $T3^d$ (*ac*)

vīśālāṃ rasataś *cāhus* tiktām uṣṇaguṇānvitām |
uṣṇāṃ ca trivṛtām āhuḥ kaṣāyāṃ rasatas tathā || 9 || iti

a vīśālāṃ] S^{11} (-$B2^d$ K^d) $Ap2^d$ $Ib1^d$ Km^d $L1^d$ $T1^d$ (?pc) $V5a^d$ $V5b^d$; vīśālaṃ $B2^d$; vīśālaṃ| $T3^d$; vīśāla S^{22} (-$Ib1^d$ $Ib2^d$) Bo^d $P4^d$ (pc); virśālāṃ K^d; vīśālā $Ib2^d$; vīśālo $L3^d$; vīśārlā $P4^d$ (ac) **rasataś**] S (-K^d) $Ap2^d$ $L1^d$ $T1^d$ (?pc) $V5a^d$ $V5b^d$; rasaṃtaś Bo^d; rasaś K^d; rasas $T3^d$ **cāhus**] S^{11} $Ap2^d$ Bo^d $L1^d$ $T1^d$ (?pc); rāhus $V5a^d$ $V5b^d$; vādus $T3^d$; *cāpi* S^{12} **b tiktām**] S (-$B2^d$ $P4^d$) $Ap2^d$ Bo^d $L1^d$ $T1^d$ (?pc) $T3^d$ $V5a^d$ $V5b^d$; tiktam $B2^d$ $P4^d$ **-guṇānvitām**] S (-$B6^d$ $Jn3^d$ $P4^d$) $Ap2^d$ Bo^d $L1^d$ $T1^d$ (?pc) $V5a^d$ $V5b^d$; [.u]guṇānvitāṃ $B6^d$; guṇānvi[mā]⟨tā⟩^{2} $T3^d$; guṇānvitaṃ $P4^d$; guṇāśviṃtāṃ $Jn3^d$ **c uṣṇāṃ**] S (-$B2^d$ $B4^d$ $Ba2^d$) $Ap2^d$ Bo^d $L1^d$ $T1^d$ (?pc) $T3^d$ $V5a^d$ $V5b^d$; uṣṇo $B4^d$ $L3^d$; uṣṇaṃ $B2^d$ $Ba2^d$ **trivṛtām**] S $L1^d$ $T1^d$ (?pc) $V5a^d$ $V5b^d$; tṛvṛtām $Ap2^d$ Bo^d $T3^d$ **āhuḥ**] S (-$V4^d$) $Ap2^d$ Bo^d $T1^d$ (?pc) $T3^d$ $V5a^d$ $V5b^d$; ā[..]huḥ $V4^d$; āhu $L1^d$ **d kaṣāyāṃ**] S (-$P4^d$) $Ap2^d$ Bo^d $T1^d$ (?pc) $T3^d$; kaṣāyā $L1^d$ $V5a^d$ $V5b^d$; kaṣāyo $P4^d$ **rasatas tathā**] S $Ap2^d$ $L1^d$ $T1^d$ (?pc) $T3^d$ $V5a^d$ $V5b^d$; rasatasvaye Bo^d **iti**] S $Ap2^d$ $T1^d$ (?pc) $V5a^d$ $V5b^d$; ti Bo^d; *om.* $L1^d$ $T3^d$

CS Vi 8.95, 2–4

śukraśoṇitaprakṛtim, kālagarbhāśayaprakṛtim, āturāhāravihāraprakṛtim, mahābhūtavikāraprakṛtiṃ ca garbhaśarīram apekṣate.

95.1 **śukra-**] K (-$P1^ś$) $B3^d$ $C5^b$ $L2^d$ M^k Q (-$Jp2^d$) R S (-$Jn3^d$); śukrā $J2^d$ $P1^ś$; śukro $Jn3^d$; ś.kra $V5a^d$; † $Jp2^d$ **-śoṇita-**] K $B3^d$ $C5^b$ $L2^d$ M^k Q (-$Jp2^d$; ²pc $T3^d$) R S; co | ṇita $T3^d$ (ac); † $Jp2^d$ **-prakṛtim kālagarbhāśaya-**] K $B3^d$ $C5^b$ $L2^d$ M^k Q (-Q^{23}) R S; *om.* $T3^d$; † $Jp2^d$ **-prakṛtim¹**] K (-$P2^d$) $C5^b$ $L2^d$ M^k Q (-Q^{23} $Ap2^d$ $V5b^d$) S^{11} (-$B2^d$ $V4^d$) Ab^d $Ib1^d$ $T1^d$; pra | kṛtiṃ $P2^d$; prakṛti $B3^d$ R (-$T1^d$) S (-Ab^d $B4^d$ $B6^d$ $Ib1^d$ $Jn3^d$ K^d) $Ap2^d$ $C6^d$ $V5b^d$; p.k.ti $V5a^d$; † Q^{23} **kāla-**] K $B3^d$ $C5^b$ $L2^d$ M^k Q (-Q^{23}) R S (-$B4^d$ Km^d); kālaṃ $B4^d$; kāṃla Km^d $L3^d$; † Q^{23} **-garbhāśaya-**] K $B3^d$ $C5^b$ $L2^d$ M^k Q (-Q^{23}) R (-$Ib3^d$) S; garbhāśraya $C3^b$; garbhārśaya $V5a^d$; garbhaśaya $Ib3^d$; † Q^{23} **-prakṛtim²**] K (-$P1^ś$) $B3^d$ $C5^b$ $L2^d$ M^k Q (-$Jp2^d$; ²pc $T3^d$) R S; prakṛtis $Jn1^d$; prattatim $T3^d$ (ac); *om.* $J2^d$ $P1^ś$; † $Jp2^d$ **āturāhāra-**] K (-$P1^ś$ $P2^d$) $C5^b$ Q (-$Ap2^d$ $C4^b$ $Jp2^d$ $P3^d$ $V5b^d$) R^{11} (-R^{31}) S^{12} (-Ab^d); ātu(rā)hāra $P2^d$; āturāhāraṃ Ab^d; āturādāra Bo^d; ātuś cāhāra S^{11} $Ap2^d$; mātuś cāhāra $B3^d$; āturālpāhāra $L2^d$; ātrāhāra M^k; ahāmahābhūta $V5a^d$ $V5b^d$; mātur āhāra R^{31} $C3^b$ $J2^d$ $P1^ś$; mātur āhārā $P3^d$; sātur āhāra $Jn2^d$; mātur a $C4^b$; † $Jp2^d$ **-vihāra-**] K $C5^b$ $L2^d$ M^k Q (-$Ap1^d$ $Jp2^d$ $V5b^d$) R S (-$B4^d$ $V4^d$); vikāra $V5a^d$ $V5b^d$; *om.* $B3^d$ $Ap1^d$ $B4^d$ $C3^b$ $L3^d$ $V4^d$; † $Jp2^d$ **-prakṛtim³**] K $B3^d$ $C5^b$ $L2^d$ M^k Q (-Q^{23} $Ap1^d$ $V1^b$) R (-$L1^d$) S (-S^{23} $B2^d$ $T2^d$); prakṛtiḥ $V5a^d$; prakṛti S^{23} $Ap1^d$ $B2^d$ $Jn2^d$ $L1^d$ $T2^d$ $T3^d$ (²pc) U^d $V1^b$; prattati $T3^d$ (ac); † $Jp2^d$ **mahābhūtavikāraprakṛtiṃ**] K (-$J3^d$) $B3^d$ $C5^b$ $L2^d$ M^k Q (-Q^{23} $V5b^d$) S^{22} Bo^d; mahābhūtavikāraprakṛti $P4^d$; mahābhūtavikāraprakṛptiṃ U^d; maṃhābhūtavikāraprakṛtiṃ Km^d; *om.* R^{11} S^{11} $J3^d$ $T3^d$ $V5a^d$ $V5b^d$; † $Jp2^d$ **2 ca**] K $C5^b$ M^k; *om.* $B3^d$ $L2^d$ Q (-$Jp2^d$) R S; † $Jp2^d$ **-śarīram**] K $B3^d$ $C5^b$ $L2^d$ M^k Q (-$Jp2^d$ $P3^d$) R S; śarīramabh $P3^d$; śarīrabh $C6^d$; śarīrām $Jn2^d$; † $Jp2^d$ **apekṣate**] K (-$J1^d$) $B3^d$ $L2^d$ M^k Q^{11} (-$C2^b$ $V5b^d$) S (-Km^d) $T1^d$ (²pc); apekṣa $J1^d$; apekṣyate Km^d; apekṣyāraṃte $T3^d$; apakṣate $Jp3^d$; api kṛte R^{22} (ac $T1^d$); avekṣate $C2^b$ $C3^b$; avekṣeta $Jn2^d$; evevekṣeta $B5^d$; avekṣet* $B1^d$; avekṣyate $C5^b$ $L1^d$; evevekṣeta $Jn1^d$; ape† $V5a^d$ $V5b^d$; *om.* Bo^d; † $Jp2^d$

CS Vi 8.96, 6

sāndratvād upacitaparipūrṇasarvāṅgāḥ.

96.1 sāndratvād] K (-Ch^{d}) $B3^{d}$ $L2^{d}$ M^{k} Q (-$Jp3^{d}$; ^{2}*pc* $T3^{d}$) R (-R^{31}) S (-$Ib1^{d}$ Km^{d}); sāndratathād $B1^{d}$; sāṃnutvād $T3^{d}$ (*ac*); sādratvād $Ib1^{d}$ Km^{d}; sārdratvād Ch^{d}; saṃdratvād U^{d}; † $B5^{d}$ $Jn1^{d}$ $Jn2^{d}$ $Jp3^{d}$ **upacita-**] K $B3^{d}$ $L2^{d}$ M^{k} Q (-$Jp3^{d}$) R^{11} (-R^{31}) S (-S^{41} $Jn3^{d}$); u(pacita) $P3^{d}$ (*vl*); upacitā $B1^{d}$; upaccitta Bo^{d}; upasvita S^{41}; udupacita $Jn3^{d}$; † $B5^{d}$ $Jn1^{d}$ $Jn2^{d}$ $Jp3^{d}$ **-paripūrṇa-**] K (*pc* $P2^{d}$) $B3^{d}$ $L2^{d}$ M^{k} Q (-$Jp3^{d}$ $V5b^{d}$) R^{11} (-$B5^{d}$) S; paripūrṇā $P2^{d}$ (*ac*); parīpūrṇaṃ $V5b^{d}$; paritūrṇa Bo^{d}; † $B5^{d}$ $Jn1^{d}$ $Jn2^{d}$ $Jp3^{d}$ **-sarvāṅgāḥ**] Q^{21} Ch^{d}; sarvagātrāḥ K (-Ch^{d}) $B3^{d}$ $L2^{d}$ M^{k} Q^{22} Q^{23} S (-S^{31} $B4^{d}$ $P4^{d}$) Bo^{d} $C3^{b}$ $L1^{d}$; sarvagātrā $B4^{d}$; sarvagātra S^{31} $B1^{d}$; sarvagotrā $P4^{d}$; sasarvagātrāḥ R^{22}; † $B5^{d}$ $Jn1^{d}$ $Jn2^{d}$ $Jp3^{d}$

CS Vi 8.135, 6f.

-citrakasomavalkaśatāvarī-

135.1 -citraka-] $B3^{d}$ $L2^{d}$ Q (-$V5b^{d}$) R S (-$B6^{d}$ $Ib2^{d}$); citraka | $B6^{d}$; cītkra $Ib2^{d}$; trika $V5a^{d}$ $V5b^{d}$; *om.* K M^{k} **-somavalka-**] $B3^{d}$ $L2^{d}$ M^{k} Q (-$C4^{b}$ $P3^{d}$ $T3^{d}$) R^{11} S $J3^{d}$; somavalkaka K (-Ch^{d} $J3^{d}$); somavalkala Ch^{d}; somava $T3^{d}$; somakalka Bo^{d}; śomavalka $P3^{d}$; yomavalka $C4^{b}$ **-śatāvarī-**] $B3^{d}$ Q^{21}; śatāvarī | $Ap1^{d}$; śatārī $T2^{d}$ (*pc*) $V5a^{d}$ $V5b^{d}$; citraka K (-A^{d}) M^{k}; citrakaṃ A^{d} $C6^{d}$; *om.* $L2^{d}$ Q^{12} R S (*ac* $T2^{d}$) $Ap2^{d}$ $P3^{d}$

Sigla of manuscripts

Scripts: ^{b} Bengali ^{d} Devanāgarī ^{k} Kannaḍa ^{ś} Śāradā

A^{d}	Alwar, RORI 2498
Ab^{d}	Ahmedabad, B.J. Institute of Learning and Research 758
$Ap1^{d}$	Alipur, Bhogilal Leherchand Institute of Indology 5283
$Ap2^{d}$	Alipur, Bhogilal Leherchand Institute of Indology 5527
$B1^{d}$	Bikaner, RORI 1566
$B2^{d}$	Bikaner, Anup Sanskrit Library 3985
$B3^{d}$	Bikaner, Anup Sanskrit Library 3986
$B4^{d}$	Bikaner, Anup Sanskrit Library 3995
$B5^{d}$	Bikaner, Anup Sanskrit Library 3996
$B6^{d}$	Bikaner, Anup Sanskrit Library 3997
$Ba1^{d}$	Baroda, Oriental Institute 12489
$Ba2^{d}$	Baroda, Oriental Institute 25034
Bo^{d}	Bombay, Asiatic Society 172

C1[b]	Calcutta, National Library RDS 101
C2[b]	Calcutta, Library of Calcutta Sanskrit College 23
C3[b]	Calcutta, Library of Calcutta Sanskrit College 24
C4[b]	Calcutta, Asiatic Society G 4474/3
C5[b]	Calcutta, Asiatic Society G 2503/1
C6[d]	Calcutta, Asiatic Society G 4391
Ca[b]	Cambridge, Trinity College Library R 15.85
Ch[d]	Chandigarh, Lal Chand Research Library 2315
Ib1[d]	Ilāhābad, G. Jha Kendriya Sanskrit Vidyapeetha 25398
Ib2[d]	Ilāhābad, G. Jha Kendriya Sanskrit Vidyapeetha 8783/87
Ib3[d]	Ilāhābad, G. Jha Kendriya Sanskrit Vidyapeetha 37089
J1[d]	Jammu, Raghunath Temple Library 3266
J2[d]	Jammu, Raghunath Temple Library 3209
J3[d]	Jammu, Raghunath Temple Library 3330
Jn1[d]	Jamnagar, Gujarat Ayurved University Library GAS 103
Jn2[d]	Jamnagar, Gujarat Ayurved University Library GAS 118
Jn3[d]	Jamnagar, Gujarat Ayurved University Library GAS 96/2
Jp1[d]	Jaipur, Maharaja Sawai Man Singh II (MSMS) Museum 2068
Jp2[d]	Jaipur, MSMS Museum 2069
Jp3[d]	Jaipur, MSMS Museum 2561
K[d]	Koṭa, RORI 1563
Km[d]	Kathmandu, NGMPP E-40553
L1[d]	London, India Office Library (IOL) Skt. MS 335
L2[d]	London, IOL Skt. MS 881
L3[d]	London, IOL Skt. MS 1445b
M[k]	Mysore, Oriental Research Institute 902
P1[ś]	Pune, Bhandarkar Oriental Research Institute (BORI) 555 of 1875–76
P2[d]	Pune, BORI 534 of 1892[sic?]–95
P3[d]	Pune, BORI 925 of 1891–95
P4[d]	Pune, Ānandāśrama 1546
T1[d]	Tübingen, Universitätsbibliothek (UB) I.458
T2[d]	Tübingen, UB I.459
T3[d]	Tübingen, UB I.460 + I.474
U[d]	Udaipur, RORI 1474
V1[b]	Varanasi, Sarasvati Bhavan Library 44842
V2[b]	Varanasi, Sarasvati Bhavan Library 108824
V3[b]	Varanasi, Sarasvati Bhavan Library 108685
V4[d]	Varanasi, Benares Hindu

	University, Gaekwad Library C3688	***V5a***^{d}	Varanasi, Sarasvati Bhavan Library 44870
		V5b^{d}	*idem.*

Signs and abbreviations in collated and edited passages

Σ	all manuscripts, except the one(s) mentioned
..	illegible *akṣara*
.	part of an illegible *akṣara*
–	missing *akṣara* indicated by the scribe
◊	blank space in a line of text with the breadth of ca. one *akṣara*
*	*halantacihna*
†	one or more witnesses do not transmit the variant under discussion due to a lacuna
[xy]	text in square brackets was deleted in the manuscript
<xy>	text in angle brackets was added in the margin of the manuscript or elsewhere
<xy>2	text added by a second hand
ab	wavy underlining indicates that the reconstructed text is uncertain. Possible alternative readings are underlined in the apparatus.
ac	(*ante correctionem*) before a correction was applied
om.	omitted
pc	(*post correctionem*) after a correction was applied
²*pc*	after a correction was applied by a second hand
rp.	(repetition) text was miscopied a second time
tp.	(transposed) text is omitted here, but occurs at a different position
vl	variant reading within a repeated passage

References

Ācārya, Yādavaśarman Trivikrama (ed.) 1922. *Maharṣiṇā Agniveśena praṇītā CarakaDṛḍhabalābhyāṃ pratisaṃskṛtā Carakasaṃhitā. Āyurvedīyagranthamālāsaṃpādakena ācāryopāhvena trivikramātmajena Yādava-Śarmaṇā saṃśodhitā.* Mumbayyāṃ: Nirṇayasāgarayantrālaya, 2nd edn.

— 1941. *Maharṣiṇā Punarvasunopadiṣṭā, tacchiṣyeṇāgniveśena praṇītā, CarakaDṛḍhabalābhyāṃ pratisaṃskṛtā Carakasaṃhitā, śrīCakrapāṇidattaviracitayā āyurvedadīpikāvyākhyayā saṃvalitā.* Mumbayyāṃ: Nirṇayasāgara Mudrāyantrālaye, 3rd edn.

Apte, Vaman Shivaram 1957–1959. *Revised and Enlarged Edition of V.S. Apte's The Practical Sanskrit-English Dictionary.* Poona: Prasad Prakashan. 3v.

Böhtlingk, Otto 1879–1889. *Sanskrit-Wörterbuch in kürzerer Fassung.* St. Petersburg: Buchdruckerei der Kaiserlichen Akademie der Wissenschaften. 7v.

Cordier, P. 1903. "Récentes découvertes de mss. médicaux sanscrits dans l'Inde (1898–1902)." *Muséon, Nouvelle Série,* **4**, 321–52. Reprinted in Roşu 1989: 539–70.

Jolly, Julius 1901. *Medicin,* vol. 3(10) of *Grundriss der indo-arischen Philologie und Altertumskunde.* Strassburg: K. J. Trübner.

Maas, Paul 1958. *Textual Criticism. Translated from the German by Barbara Flower.* Oxford: Clarendon Press.

Maas, Philipp A. 2009. "Towards a Critical Edition of the Carakasaṃhitā Vimānasthāna – First Results." *Indian Journal of History of Science,* **44(2)**, 163–85.

— 2010a. "Computer Aided Stemmatics – The Case of Fifty-Two Text Versions of Carakasaṃhitā Vimānasthāna 8.67–157." *Wiener Zeitschrift für die Kunde Südasiens,* **52–53**, 63–119.

— 2010b. "On What Became of the Carakasaṃhitā After

Dṛḍhabala's Revision." *eJournal of Indian Medicine*, **3**, 1–22.

Meulenbeld, Gerrit Jan 1999–2002. *A History of Indian Medical Literature*, vol. XV of *Groningen Oriental Studies*. Groningen: E. Forsten. 5v.

Monier-Williams, Monier, E. Leumann, and C. Cappeller 1899. *A Sanskrit–English Dictionary Etymologically and Philologically Arranged, New Edition*. Oxford: Clarendon Press. 1970 reprint.

Preisendanz, Karin, Cristina Pecchia, and Philipp A. Maas (eds.) in preparation. Text of the Carakasaṃhitā Vimānasthāna as critically edited by the "Philosophy and Medicine in Early Classical India" projects at the University of Vienna.

Roşu, Arion 1989. *Un demi-siècle de recherches āyurvédiques. Gustave Liétard et Palmyr Cordier: Travaux sur l'histoire de la médecine indienne*. Paris: Institut de Civilisation Indienne.

Senagupta, Narendranātha and Balāicandra Senagupta (eds.) 1927. *Caraka-saṃhitā. mahāmuninā bhagavatĀgniveśena praṇītā maharṣiCarakeṇa pratisaṃskṛtā. Carakacaturānana-śrīmacCakrapāṇidattapraṇītayā Āyurvedadīpikākhyaṭīkayā mahāmahopādhyāya-śrīGaṅgādharakaviratnakavirājaviracitayā Jalpakalpatarusamākhyayā ṭīkayā ca samalaṅkṛtā. kavirāja śrīNarendranātha Senaguptena kavirāja śrīBalāicandra Senaguptena ca sampāditā saṃśodhitā prakāśitā ca.* Kalikātānagaryyāṃ: Dhanvantari Steam Machine Press.

Timpanaro, Sebastiano 2005. *The Genesis of Lachmann's Method, Edited and Translated [from Italian into English] by Glenn W. Most*. Chicago and London: University of Chicago Press. Original Italian edition, *La genesi del metodo del Lachmann*, Padova 1971.

West, Martin L. 1973. *Textual Criticism and Editorial Technique applicable to Greek and Latin Texts*. Stuttgart: Teubner.

3

Karin Preisendanz

Logic, Debate and Epistemology in Ancient Indian Medical Science: An Investigation into the History and Historiography of Indian Philosophy Part I

1.1 In the introduction to his *Comparative History of World Philosophy*, the philosopher Ben-Ami Scharfstein justifies his view that there are only three great philosophical traditions – the Indian, the Chinese and the European – and

Research on this paper was generously supported by the FWF (Austrian Science Fund), Projects No. P14451-SPR ("Debate in the Context of the History of Indian Medicine"), P17300-G03 ("Philosophy and Medicine in Early Classical India") and P19866–G15 ("Philosophy and Medicine in Early Classical India II"). For further information on these projects, their aims and results, see the website of the most recent project at `http://www.istb.univie.ac.at/caraka` (viewed March 2011). Thanks to the cooperation and kind assistance of many institutions in India and Europe, copies of some fifty MSS of the *Vimānasthāna* of the *Carakasaṃhitā* have become available to the projects. I am immensely grateful to all of them, especially to the institutions that own the MSS explicitly referred to in the present contribution (*Ca*^{b}, *L1*^{d}, *L2*^{d}, *T1*^{d}, *T2*^{d}, *T3*^{d}, *V2*^{b}, *V3*^{b}): the Trinity College Library, Cambridge, the British Library, London, the Universitätsbibliothek (University Library) Tübingen, and the Sarasvati Bhavana Library, Varanasi. This is a slightly revised, augmented and updated version of a paper that was previously published in unauthorized, deprecated form in *Indian Journal of History of Science* 44,2 (2009) 261–312. I am grateful to Eli Franco for his thorough reading of earlier versions of this paper, and to Albrecht Wezler for his comments on the *IJHS* paper.

treats *inter alia* the question of what he considers as "philosophical" in the context of this book. According to him, a tradition can be called philosophical first of all to the extent that the persons associated with it express its contents in the form of basic principles and inferences rationally derived from these principles. Furthermore, a tradition may be called "philosophical" to the extent that its followers justify these contents with rational arguments and defend them vis-à-vis the followers of other, rival traditions, or attack their positions, again by means of rational arguments. Finally, a tradition is also to be considered philosophical to the extent that its adherents understand and explain in which manner they strive for rational practice, that is, to the extent that they explicate their methods of argumentation and justification. The two central characteristics of a philosophical tradition are thus logic and disputation or debate, i.e., characteristics which are usually not found in so-called wisdom traditions; the latter comprise elaborate, but purely religious traditions, mythological traditions or traditions of practical intelligence.[1]

1.2 In the classical philosophical traditions of India in general, the two components of logic and debate are closely intertwined from the historical point of view. This is especially obvious in the case of the Nyāyaśāstra, the expert body of knowledge concerned with "logic," and its authoritative foundational work, the *Nyāyasūtra*.[2] As is well

---

[1]See Scharfstein 1998, especially pp. 1–4 and 21–33. The introduction to Scharfstein 1998 is also found, with slight variations, in Scharfstein 1997.

[2]The word *nyāya* is frequently translated as "logic." However, it is often forgotten that its meaning is first of all "right way" or "right manner." From this the meaning "suitable method" is derived, i.e., a method or rule which lets one reliably achieve one's aims. According to Pāṇini's (P)

known, the basic metaphysical tenets of the Nyāyaśāstra are closely related to a tradition of philosophy of nature whose various teachings are preserved in some early philosophical tracts found in the Mokṣadharma section of the *Mahābhārata*. Similar tenets appear as the ontological foundations of early classical Ayurveda and form the main subject of the classical Vaiśeṣika tradition. In the case of Nyāya epistemology and eristics, which according to the testimony of the *Nyāyasūtra* were the initial foci of interest for the thinkers of this tradition, striking and interesting parallels are to be found in the *Carakasaṃhitā*.

The issue of the historical relationship between the epistemological and eristic teachings transmitted in the *Carakasaṃhitā*, on the one hand, and the epistemology and eristics of classical Nyāya, on the other hand, is the central topic of this paper, with an initial focus on eristics. This focus can be justified by means of the assumption that in the Indian context, where the learned exchange of ideas and opinions as well as disputation in the broadest sense of the word were practised from early on, the theoretical concern with the principles and elements of scholarly debate contributed considerably to the development of epistemology,

---

sūtra 3.3.37 (*parinyor nīṇor dyūtābhreṣayoḥ*), the suffix *ghañ* (see P 3.3.16), which refers to the instrument (*karaṇa*) or substratum (*adhikaraṇa*) (see P 3.3.120, with P 3.3.118 and 117), is added to the verbal root $\sqrt{i}$ in combination with the preverb *ni-* in the sense of "non-deviation/aberration." *nyāya* is thus the means used to arrive at a certain goal without fail or deviation, i.e., the proper way or right manner, and may consequently also refer to a method or rule/maxim. Similarly, the word *pariṇāya*, literally "the means by which one moves [tokens or figures] around [in a board game]," refers to a move in such a game. Eventually, the word *nyāya* came to be used to specifically refer to methodical and systematic thinking, that is, coherent and correct logical reflection and argumentation. See Preisendanz 2010 for further details on this development. For the sake of brevity only, I will use the expression "logic" in the following.

including logic. More precisely, the consideration of the demonstration or statement of proof, central to any debate, can safely be assumed to have led to in-depth reflection on the foundations and means of knowledge, and thus to the development of theories of perception and logical theories. Beyond the immediate context of public or semi-public debates, the ancient Indian thinkers and scholars obviously applied the ascertained means of knowledge in their own methodical reflections on doctrinal issues and their further development. This happened in the context of the rigorous examination of the argumentative and factual coherence and appropriateness (*yukti*) of doctrinal issues, in the process of the "turning around" (*tarka*) of these issues, that is, in the process of reasoning about them, and in the course of examining and corroborating them by means of reasons (*hetu*). In the course of the further development and systematization of Indian philosophy and its individual traditions, and especially in the context of the polemical dialogue with rival traditions, the epistemological foundations became themselves an important topic of reflection and contention.

2.1 After this brief sketch of the general background, I would now like to turn to the *Carakasaṃhitā* (*CS*). The first instalment of this foundational work was edited by Gangadhar Kaviraj and published in 1868.[3] Gangadhar Kaviraj (1798–1885) was a learned Bengali physician and chief reviver of the Ayurvedic tradition in the modern period who wrote about eighty works, original and commentaries, in different areas of Sanskrit learning;[4] in his

[3]For some notes on the earliest edition of the *Carakasaṃhitā*, see Appendix, p. 123 below.

[4]On Gangadhar Kaviraj see Chakravarti 1929–1930: 254 f. and Gupta 1976: 371 f.; more recently, a small monograph was devoted to him

editio princeps of the *Carakasaṃhitā*, he supplemented the classical text with his own extensive Sanskrit commentary *Jalpakalpataru*.[5] However, the text was published only step by step, and communication between India and Europe took its time. The first Western scholar who turned his attention to selected aspects of the *Carakasaṃhitā* relevant to the present topic, the German Indologist Rudolf Roth (1821–1895), thus still had to rely on manuscripts for the pertinent passages. Roth was not only professor of Indology, but from 1856 onwards also director of the library of the University of Tübingen for which he acquired a considerable number of manuscripts from India.[6] A Devanāgarī-script manuscript of the *Carakasaṃhitā* was obtained by Roth through the good offices of August Hoernle,[7] a scholar who was to become an important pi-

by Chattopadhyay (Chattopadhyay 1995, mainly relating to the manuscripts of Gangadhar's works preserved in the library of the Calcutta Sanskrit College). See also Meulenbeld 1999: IB, p. 287 f.

[5]On the different editions of the *Jalpakalpataru*, see again Meulenbeld 1999: IB, p. 287 f.

[6]See von Stietencron 2003: 77 f.; see also Zeller 2003: 111, with n. 39, on an acquisition trip to India by Roth's former student Richard Garbe, and on Aurel Stein, another of Roth's students, who send some birchbark manuscripts from Kashmir to Roth still in the final year of Roth's life.

[7]MS I. 458, no. 141 in Garbe 1899: 62 f. ($T1^d$). This MS contains many marginalia and corrections by a second hand, which is most probably that of Roth himself; see Preisendanz 2007: 635, n. 36, and Pecchia 2010: 154f. for further details. In one case (*CS Vi* 8.144) a note with variant readings on *āmrāsthyambaṣṭhakī* is clearly relying on the reading in a *Carakasaṃhitā* MS of the India Office Library, London (Sanskrit MSS 335 and 1535, no. 2637 f. in Eggeling 1896: 923–25) ($L1^d$), where during the years 1843–1845, immediately after he had received his Ph.D. degree, Roth did extensive research (see von Stietencron 2003: 80 and Zeller 2003: 92). He may have copied this MS, or extracts from it, already at this time, as he did with many other Sanskrit MSS preserved in Paris, London and Oxford (see von Stietencron, loc. cit.) (for a different scenario,

oneering authority in the Western study of classical Indian medicine; Roth could furthermore use a Bengali-script manuscript which is still preserved at Trinity College, Cambridge.[8] He was obviously intrigued by the *Carakasaṃhitā* because in this work medical knowledge is embedded within a wider cultural, social and philosophical context. Thus, in 1872 he translated a substantial portion from the beginning of the eighth chapter of the *Vimānasthāna* (*Vi*) of the *Carakasaṃhitā*,[9] namely, the passages that deal with the preliminaries of choosing the medical career and with the choice of a teacher in this field, and then treat the general requirements and rules for studying and teaching, including the selection of a student by a teacher and the former's ritual initiation into studenthood.[10]

2.2 In this pedagogical context, the topic of debate or colloquy (*sambhāṣā*) is introduced inasmuch as debate is considered a didactic means to be employed beneficially in medical training and a useful tool in the continuing refinement and improvement of medical knowledge.[11] Peaceful

---

see Pecchia 2010: 155). A further MS of the *Carakasaṃhitā* owned by the University Library, Tübingen, was copied later, in 1873, commissioned and procured by Hoernle in the same year (MS I. 459, no. 142, in Garbe 1899: 63) ($T2^d$). Still another one, which is incomplete (MSS I. 460 and 474, nos. 143 and 152 in Garbe 1899: 63 and 65 f.) ($T3^d$) and written by the same hand, may also have reached Tübingen at this time, that is, only after Roth had already written his seminal paper published in 1872.

[8] MS no. R. 15. 85 in Aufrecht 1869: 21–24 (Ca^b). See Preisendanz 2007: 635, n. 37, for further details.

[9] *CS Vi* 8.1–26 and, as a conclusion written in comparable style, 67 (see below, p. 74).

[10] See Roth 1872. On the initiation of the medical student according to Caraka, see Preisendanz 2007.

[11] *CS Vi* 8.15. On the entire section *Vi* 8.15–26 see the translation and extensive annotation, interpretation and discussion in Kang 2003.

colloquies (*sandhāyasambhāṣā*)[12] are distinguished from hostile colloquies (*vigṛhyasambhāṣā*),[13] terms and notions clearly related to the concepts of *sandhi* and *vigraha* which are well known from Kauṭilya's *Arthaśāstra*[14] and related literature.[15] And indeed, the relevant passage, in its practical tone and refreshingly idiomatic style, suggests that debate was also practised, even in a ruthless manner, to resolve conflicts arising from the competition between rival traditions or schools of physicians, more precisely, to neutralize adherents of other traditions as well as outright quacks, by means of successfully conducted debates on medical topics and thus to counteract (un)professional competition.

2.3 Following almost fifty years after the publication of Roth's paper in a German-language Orientalists' journal, the *Carakasaṃhitā* prominently appeared on the stage of non-medical scholarly literature in Satis Chandra Vidyabhusana's *History of Indian Logic. Ancient, Mediaeval and Modern Schools*, which was published in 1921 from Calcutta just after the death of the great *savant*.[16] Vidyabhusana (1870–1920) was a true pioneer in the investigation of the literature and history of Indian logic. He was aware of an

---

[12]The peaceful colloquy is also called "favourable/agreeable colloquy" (*anulomasambhāṣā*) (see the conclusion of *CS Vi* 8.17).

[13]See *CS Vi* 8.16 and 18.

[14]See *sandhi* ("alliance," "treaty") and *vigraha* ("conflict") in the context of the complex of six expedients or policies (*ṣāḍguṇya*) of a ruler according to *AS* 7, especially 7.1; further on this see Scharfe 1989: 206–9. See also n. 32 below.

[15]See, e.g., *PT* III, first story; the six expedients are listed p. 135, 2f. and subsequently discussed, with a focus on *sandhi* and *vigraha*, by King Meghavarṇa's five ministers. Cp. also the names of the third and fourth section of the *Hitopadeśa*.

[16]See Vidyabhusana 1921: 25–35. For a brief historical placement and appreciation of this book, see Randle 1926: 84f.

amazingly broad range of sources and often was the first modern scholar to point them out; his references are not only to Brahminical philosophical literature, but also to Indian Buddhist philosophical literature, most of which was then only available in Tibetan translation, and to philosophical literature of the Jains. In 1909, Vidyabhusana edited for the first time the oldest preserved Jain work on logic, the *Nyāyāvatāra* by Siddhasena Divākara, who may have been a younger contemporary of Dharmakīrti.[17] The Tibetan text of Dharmakīrti's *Nyāyabindu*, the well-known manual on epistemology and especially logic composed by this important philosopher of the so-called Buddhist epistemological–logical tradition, was also edited by him for the first time in 1917; he further prepared a bilingual index (Sanskrit – Tibetan) to this work, in order to facilitate and stimulate the investigation of the Indian Buddhist epistemological–logical works preserved only in Tibetan translation.[18] Moreover, Vidyabhusana edited and translated the text of the *Nyāyasūtra* (1909).

In his *History of Indian Logic*, Vidyabhusana collected evidence for the early history of Indian logic, whose very foundation under the name of *ānvīkṣikī* he ascribes, in partial reverence for the tradition, to the sage Medhātithi

---

[17]See Balcerowicz 2001: iii–xxxiv, who dates the *Nyāyāvatāra* between 620 and 800.

[18]Further Buddhist works in Tibetan translation edited by Vidyabhusana, partly with translation, are the *Prātimokṣasūtra* and the *Lalitavistara* (twelfth chapter) (both 1912). Moreover, Vidyabhusana edited the *Sragdharātārāstotra* of Sarvajñamitra (1908) and two of the songs of Milarepa (1912), both widely spread in Nepal. With his edition of the Tibetan translation of the *Amarakośa* (1911–1912) Vidyabhusana also turned to non-Buddhist literature in Tibetan translation. Little known is his monograph on Tibetan scrolls and images from Gyantse (1905), and his articles on historical topics.

Gautama.[19] In this context, Vidyabhuysana refers to various passages of the *Sūtrasthāna* and *Vimānasthāna* of the *Carakasaṃhitā*, namely, passages that he perceives as summaries or reproductions of what he styles "the principal doctrines of Ānvīkṣikī;" only a few technical terms, he says, may have been introduced by the redactor Caraka.[20] This Ānvīkṣikī or "investigating [science]" was – according to Vidyabhusana – later on embodied or assimilated in the *Nyāyasūtra* by the philosopher Akṣapāda,[21] when the science of syllogism or inference, the Nyāyaśāstra, had already begun to develop as a special sub-discipline within the *ānvīkṣikī* and obtained a name of its own; this Nyāyaśāstra had even been shaped to a certain extent by Akṣapāda himself.[22] The assimilation of the Ānvīkṣikī, or rather the Nyāyaśāstra, in the *Nyāyasūtra* supposedly happened less than a century after Caraka had achieved the redaction of Agniveśa's teachings, an event which Vidyabhusana dates towards the end of the first century.[23] The described process resulted – in Vidyabhusana's view – in the emergence of the "first regular work on the Nyāyaśāstra",[24] i.e., the formation of the systematic philosophical tradition of Nyāya (see Figure 3.1).

---

[19]See Vidyabhusana 1921: 17–21. In the introduction to his 1913 edition and translation of the *Nyāyasūtra*, Vidyabhusana still identifies Gotama/Gautama and Akṣapāda (Vidyabhusana 1909: ii–xi). Nanda Lal Sinha, in his introduction to his revised edition of Vidyabhusana's edition and translation, expresses harsh criticism of this change in opinion (Vidyabhusana 1930: v–ix).

[20]See Vidyabhusana 1921: 25–35, quotation at p. 25. On the items possibly inserted by Caraka according to Vidyabhusana see n. 51 below.

[21]See Vidyabhusana 1921: 26 and 50.

[22]See Vidyabhusana 1921: 39–45, especially p. 40.

[23]See Vidyabhusana 1921: 27 and 50.

[24]See Vidyabhusana 1921: 46.

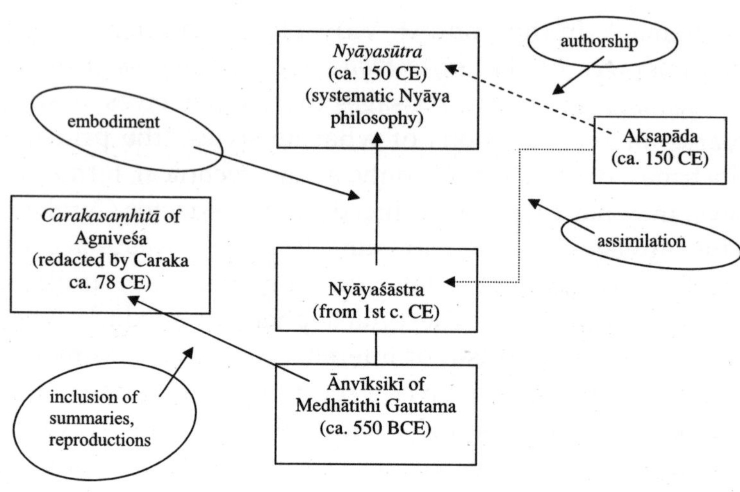

Figure 3.1: The Development of Nyāya According to Vidyabhusana

3 Let us now take a look at the passages of the *Carakasaṃhitā* adduced by Vidyabhusana as the basis for his hypothesis. Vidyabhusana himself structured the material presented in them according to three heads; in his own words and supplied with Sanskrit key-words, they are

1. the aggregate of resources for the accomplishment of an action (*kāryābhinirvṛtti*),
2. the standard of examination (*parīkṣā*), and
3. the method of debate (*sambhāṣā* or *vāda-vidhi*).[25]

Of these, the first topic[26] is not considered to have been part of Medhātithi's Ānvīkṣikī by Vidyabhusana; thus, only the second and third topics are of immediate relevance to the present issue. Because in Vidyabhusana's opinion the

[25]See Vidyabhusana 1921: 26.

[26]See also n. 34 below.

method of debate was the principal topic of Ānvīkṣikī,[27] I would like to turn to it first.

3.1.1 Vidyabhusana first summarizes in a close paraphrase the section on the purpose, merit and characteristics of a scholarly colloquy (*sambhāṣā*). This section involves the typological classification of colloquies already referred to above (see p. 68) and of their components in the broadest sense of the word, namely, the two participants and the attending assembly (*parṣad*); it also offers various practical advice to the disputants, inclusive of the advance manipulation of the assembly (see Table 3.1).[28]

Vidyabhusana then continues with an enumerative exposition of the altogether forty-four relevant points or topics (*pada*) to be understood for the purpose of knowing the way of disputation (*vāda*).[29] These relevant topics, presented by Vidyabhusana under the slightly misleading term "categories," are listed immediately after the section on colloquies briefly analyzed above.[30] Subsequently, they are characterized, further classified and exemplified, often with reference to medical topics and issues belonging to the realm of philosophy of nature.[31]

3.1.2 The section on disputation (*vāda*) appears to be composed in a strikingly different, austere style of language and with a more systematic mind when compared to the preceding lively section on colloquies (*sambhāṣā*). From a

---

[27]See Vidyabhusana 1921: 27.

[28]See Vidyabhusana 1921: 28–31 on *CS Vi* 8.15–26. See also the summaries in Solomon 1976: 74–77 and Frauwallner 1984: 68f.

[29]See *CS Vi* 8.27 and 66, and Vidyabhusana 1921: 31–35.

[30]See *CS Vi* 8.27, quoted in n. 40 below.

[31]See *CS Vi* 8.28–65.

[32]The types are: *pravara* (superior), *pratyavara* (inferior) and *sama* (equal); see *CS Vi* 8.19. Also in the context of the *Arthaśāstra's* six ex-

diverse usefulness of colloquies	15
two types of colloquies; three types of opponents (*para*);[32] two types of assemblies (*parṣad*)	16–21
admonitory verses on hostile colloquies	22–23
advance manipulation of the assembly and the setting of limits for the disputation (*vāda*)	24–26

Table 3.1: The Section on Colloquies (*sambhāṣā*) in *Carakasaṃhitā Vimānasthāna* (8.15–26)

stylistic point of view, this latter section may even be perceived as concluded with text segment 67, which occurs in a similar style immediately after the more rigorous exposition of the forty-four relevant topics.[33] Segment 67 is harmoniously followed by an extensive excursus – actually taking up the sizeable rest of the chapter – which is basically written in the same style and occasioned by the concluding reference to the significance of debate for successful medical practice. This excursus may be entitled "How to act successfully" and starts out from the presentation of

pedients, which include *sandhi* and *vigraha*, the other/opponent kings are classified into three types: *sama* (equal), *jyāyas* (superior) and *hīna* (inferior); see especially AŚ 7.3.1–20.

[33]See *CS* (crit. ed.) *Vi* 8.67: *vādas tu khalu bhiṣajāṃ vartamāno vartetāyurveda eva, nānyatra. tatra hi vākyaprativākyavistarāḥ kevalāś copapattayaḥ sarvādhikaraṇeṣu. tāḥ sarvāḥ samyag avekṣyāvekṣya vākyaṃ brūyāt, nāprakṛtakam aśāstrakam aparīkṣitam asādhakam ākulam ajñāpakaṃ vā. sarvaṃ ca hetumad brūyāt. hetumanto hy akaluṣāḥ sarva eva vādavigrahāś cikitsite kāraṇabhūtāḥ praśastabuddhivardhakatvāt; sarvārambhasiddhiṃ hy āvahaty anupahatā buddhiḥ.* (Wavy underlining marks uncertain readings.) Even though the text of the *Carakasaṃhitā* quoted in the present paper is the text as established in the new critical edition, the numbering of text segments here still follows that in Trikamji's edition.

enumeration of forty-four topics (*padas*)	27
their characterization, sub-classification and exemplification	28–65
conclusion concerning the forty-four *padas*	66
concluding remarks on disputation/debate as such (*vāda*)	67
"How to act successfully" (ten topical complexes [*prakaraṇa*] / ten items to be examined [*parīkṣya*])	68–151

Table 3.2: The Section on Disputation (*vāda*) in *CS Vi* 8 (27–66) and the Continuation of the Chapter

a scientific methodology involving ten topical complexes (*prakaraṇa*) that lead to success in acting in general and should be known by physicians before they embark on their task, so that they can accomplish it without overly great effort.[34] The general methodology comprising these ten topical complexes as something to be examined (*parīkṣya*) is then once more recommended to physicians[35] and its details expounded in the form of answers to nine questions – posed by a physician or lay-person to a physician – regarding this methodology when applied by a physician with a view to the five-fold therapy (*pañcakarma*)[36] (see Table 3.2).

The obviously composite nature of the entire passage on debate is also reflected in a corresponding change in terminology for the main issue, namely, the shift from *sambhāṣā*

[34]See *CS Vi* 68–78. This is the topic called *kāryābhinirvṛtti* in Vidyabhusana 1921: 26 and 27.

[35]See *CS Vi* 8.79.

[36]See *CS Vi* 8.80–151. For a detailed topical and structural analysis of *CS Vi* 8 see Preisendanz 2007: Appendix 3.

("colloquy") to *vāda*, literally: "talk," but also referring to "discussion" or "disputation".[37] This shift is prepared in the closing text segments of what I will henceforth briefly call the "*sambhāṣā* section," inasmuch as in these segments the word *vāda* is already introduced.[38] It may have been used here in its general, non-terminological sense and thus be part of the original wording of these segments; alternatively, the word may have been intended as a technical term and therefore be the trace of a redactional effort to smoothen the shift. The diverging term *vāda* also appears in the concluding text segment 67 already referred to above (p. 74) which comes after what I will now call the "*vāda* section." In the summarizing verses of the chapter, the terminological discrepancy relating to the two sections is properly reflected.[39]

3.1.3 After this overview of the relevant passage in the context of *CS Vi* 8, I would like to take a look at the *vāda* section, in order to clarify and evaluate Vidyabhusana's reasoning regarding his reconstruction of the development of Indian logic and the Nyāya tradition. Obviously, the list of forty-four *padas*[40] shows a considerable closeness in terminology

---

[37] On different terminologies concerning debate and its various classifications on the basis of the evidence of *CS Vi* 8 and the *Nyāyasūtra*, see Preisendanz 2000 [2001]: 232 f. See furthermore Kang 2003: 17–42 where additional material is considered and discussed.

[38] See *CS Vi* 8.24–26.

[39] See *CS Vi* 8.152 (*sambhāṣāvidhi*) and 153 (*vādamārgapadāni*). Prets (2010: 71) mistakenly refers to the section concerned with the forty-four relevant topics as the *sambhāṣāvidhi*.

[40] See *CS Vi* 8.27 (crit. ed.): *imāni khalu padāni vādamārgajñānārtham adhigamyāni: vādo dravyaṃ guṇāḥ karma sāmānyaṃ viśeṣaḥ samavāyaḥ pratijñā sthāpanā pratiṣṭhāpanā hetur upanayo nigamanam uttaraṃ dṛṣṭāntaḥ siddhāntaḥ śabdaḥ pratyakṣam aupamyam aitihyam anumānaṃ saṃśayaḥ prayojanaṃ savyabhicāraṃ jijñāsā vyavasāyo 'rthaprāptiḥ saṃbhavo 'nuyojyam*

– also observable in some of the subsequent characterizations of individual items – to the sixteen dialectical–eristic items, listed in the *Nyāyasūtra* (*NS*) and called "relevant matters" (*padārtha*) in classical Nyāya[41] even though, as has been stressed by Halbfass,[42] the word *padārtha* is not yet used in the *Nyāyasūtra*. Together with their characterizations, these items form the programmatic and methodological backbone of the Nyāya philosophical tradition as presented in the core stratum of the *Nyāyasūtra*. Thus, Vidyabhusana felt justified to claim the list of *pada*s in the *Carakasaṃhitā* to be originally an essential part of the Ānvīkṣikī ascribed by him to Medhātithi Gautama and considered to have evolved into the Nyāyaśāstra, which is the foundation of the *Nyāyasūtra*. In a "crude form," as he phrases it, this ancient list is preserved in the *Carakasaṃhitā*; however, it also found its way into the *Nyāyasūtra* after having been "pruned" by Akṣapāda, resulting in the classical list of sixteen *padārtha*s.[43] According to Vidyabhusana, this process of pruning of the ancient topics and their "assimilation" in the *Nyāyasūtra* by Akṣapāda went together with Akṣapāda's systematization of the concept of means of knowledge and his introduction of the scheme of the five parts of a syllogism, as well as of the examination of other, rival positions (see Figure 3.2).[44]

ananuyojyam anuyogaḥ pratyanuyogo vākyadoṣo vākyapraśaṃsā chalam ahetavo 'tītakālam upālambhaḥ parihāraḥ pratijñāhānir abhyanujñā hetvantaram arthāntaraṃ nigrahasthānam iti.

[41]See especially *NS* 1.1.1: *pramāṇaprameyasaṃśayaprayojanadṛṣṭāntasiddhāntāvayavatarkanirṇayavādajalpavitaṇḍāhetvābhāsajātinigrahasthānānāṃ tattvajñānān niḥśreyasādhigamaḥ.*

[42]See Halbfass 1992: 85, n. 39.

[43]See Vidyabhusana 1921: 26. For a brief characterization of this hypothesis, see also Filliozat 1990: 43.

[44]See Vidyabhusana 1921: 49f.

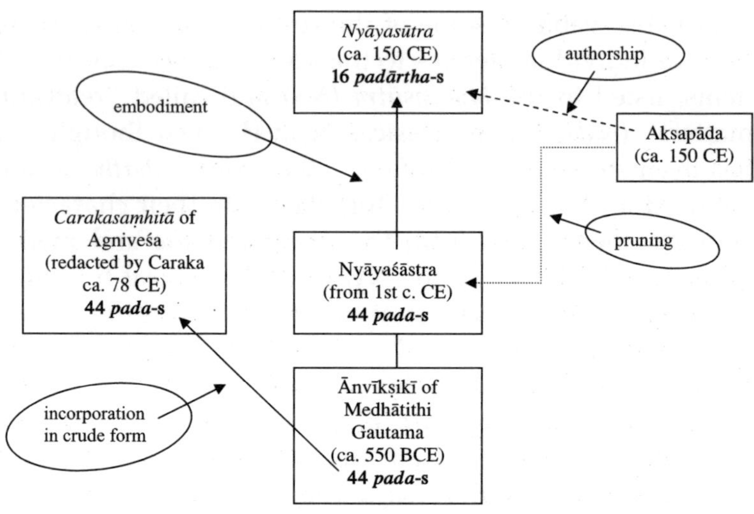

Figure 3.2: The History of the List of Forty-four *pada*s According to Vidyabhusana

A comparative and correlative historical exposition of all the topics involved was not presented by Vidyabhusana. Due to the complexity of the issues, the historical uncertainties and the many interpretative problems, such an exposition cannot be meaningfully attempted in the context of this paper; only a few exemplary cases will be briefly alluded to or presented below. For my present purpose a rough typological–analytical survey of Caraka's crucial list of *pada*s very well suffices and may also throw some new light on it, even without consideration of the characterizations or descriptions and exemplifications provided for each item in the text segments subsequent to the list.[45]

[45]See *CS Vi* 8.28–65. For a paraphrase see Solomon 1976: 78–86. A comparative survey with historical interpretation is also provided in Frauwallner 1984: 70–81 and Oberhammer 1963: 73–75. On the nature of

1	disputation (*vāda*)
2–7	basic ontological terms/categories (*dravya, guṇa, karman, sāmānya, viśeṣa, samavāya*)
8–16	terms relating to the structure of argumentation and types of statements in a disputation

Table 3.3: The Forty-four Topics (*CS Vi* 8.27) I

3.1.4 In an overall tentatively systematic manner, the list presents, next to some ontological terms, a number of more or less technical terms relating to eristic debate, i.e., disputation (*vāda*), as well as to rhetorics and epistemology. Disputation itself is the very first item, followed by six ontological terms known from classical Vaiśeṣika and a group of terms loosely connected with the structure of argumentation and important types of statements in a disputation (see Table 3.3).

The first six terms of the latter group of terms, namely, *pratijñā, sthāpanā, pratiṣṭhāpanā, hetu, upanaya*[46] and *nigamana*, concern the most essential steps to be taken by a speaker to communicate his theses convincingly; only one of the listed steps, the *pratiṣṭhāpanā*, may be a step taken by his opponent.[47] The demonstration or statement of proof (*hetu*) is central among these steps (see Table 3.4).

the explanatory text segments, see n. 118 below and, for a specific case, p. 119 below.

[46]On the characterization and explication of *upanaya* in *CS Vi* 8.31f. see Oetke 1994: 81f., n. 48, and 149f., n. 84.

[47]On *sthāpanā* and *pratiṣṭhāpanā*, and their relation to *nigamana* in the *Carakasaṃhitā*, see Oetke 1994: 47–50, 61 and 226; on their relation to the five elements of argumentation, Oberhammer 1963: 79–81.

8	thesis (*pratijñā*) (1)
9	setting up one's thesis (*sthāpanā*) (2)
10	setting up the counter-thesis (*pratiṣṭhāpanā*) (3)
11	demonstrations / statements of proof (*hetu*) (4)
12	application (*upanaya*) (5)
13	conclusion (*nigamana*) (6)

Table 3.4: Terms Relating to the Structure of Argumentation and Types of Statements in a Disputation I

Let me briefly add here that in the editions of the *Carakasaṃhitā* following Gangadhar Kaviraj's edition with his own commentary *Jalpakalpataru* – which include Jadavji Trikamji's edition that has attained the status of the standard text of the *Carakasaṃhitā* in the modern period[48] – another item, *dṛṣṭānta*, occurs between *hetu* and *upanaya*.[49] However, according to the evidence of the manuscripts available to the projects on the critical edition of the *Vimānasthāna*,[50] *dṛṣṭānta* has its "regular place" before the last term of the following sub-group, namely, *siddhānta*. This group of three terms also refers to statements – or the con-

[48]There are three editions of this book published by the Nirnaya Sagar Press: first edition 1933, second edition 1935, third edition 1941. To my knowledge, the various modern reprints are produced from the third, augmented edition.

[49]See also Prets 2010: 69 on this discrepancy and on the editions which read as in the critical edition.

[50]See acknowledgement note p. 63 above. See also Prets 2010: 73–76 on the evidence of some of the MSS used in the context of the pilot project on critically editing the *Vimānasthāna* 8 (P14451–SPR), of Cakrapāṇidatta's commentary and Gangadhar Kaviraj's *Mṛtyuñjayasaṃhitā*. Prets' statements and observations on the text genealogy and the stemmatic relationship of the MSS are now largely obsolete (see also Prets 2010: 85); the reader is referred to the more recent publications by Maas, i.e., his contribution to the present volume, as well as Maas 2010a and 2010b.

14	replies (*uttara*) (7)
15	generally acknowledged matters (*dṛṣṭānta*) (8)
16	fixed positions / presuppositions (*siddhānta*) (9)

Table 3.5: Terms Relating to the Structure of Argumentation and Types of Statements in a Disputation II

tent of statements – that must have had their structurally determined place in a disputation (see Table 3.5).[51]

3.1.5.1 Subsequently, as shown in Table 3.6, the list of *pada*s switches to epistemological terms relevant to disputation, terms denoting cognitive–psychological concepts obviously of relevance in a disputation, and terms somehow relating to the truth of statements uttered in a disputation.

17–21	epistemological terms
22–26	terms denoting cognitive–psychological concepts
27–32	terms relating to the truth of statements in a disputation

Table 3.6: The Forty-four Topics (*CS Vi* 8.27) II

The first group comprises five items which elsewhere in early classical philosophical sources can be found subsumed under the well-known concept of means of valid cognition or means of knowledge (*pramāṇa*).[52] In Table 3.7

[51]Vidyabhusana (1921: 27) considers that the whole group of nine terms starting with *pratijñā* and ending with *siddhānta* may have been inserted by Caraka into the *vādamārga* when he redacted the Saṃhitā in the first century CE because Medhātithi Gautama may not have been familiar with these terms in their technical sense.

[52]On the sources of knowledge as presented in *CS Vi* 8 and other related early sources, see Kang 2007: 64–84.

17	verbal testimony (*śabda*) (1)
18	sense perception (*pratyakṣa*) (2)
19	comparison/analogy (*aupamya*) (3)
20	oral tradition (*aitihya*) (4)
21	inference (*anumāna*) (5)

Table 3.7: Epistemological Terms

I have adopted as original the order of these items in the list that is found in all MSS of the Kashmiri recension of the *Carakasaṃhitā* (K) as well as almost all MSS belonging to the Bengali branch of the Eastern recension of the text (Q [-Q[31]]);[53] the remaining MSS show the order adopted in Trikamji's standard edition.[54] The order of the subsequent text segments where the individual items are characterized or described and exemplified (Vi 8.38–42) corresponds to the original sequence established here, except in the minor sub-group of MSS Q[31] and in MS Ca[b].

The very appearance of these items in the present context suggests that the thinkers we encounter here were

[53]MS *L2*[d] (owned by the India Office Library, London, Sanskrit MS 881, no. 2640 in Eggeling 1896: 926 f.) also has this sequence. Q[31] comprises two MSS owned by the Sarasvati Bhavana Library, Varanasi: *V2*[b] (acc. no. 107465, no. 108824 in DCSSUV) and *V3*[b] (acc. no. 108221, no. 108685 in DCSSUV). *V2*[b] was personally written, partly with a commentary, by Gangadhar Kaviraj in *śaka* 1760, i.e., 1838/1839 AD; see also p. 21 f. of the paper by Cristina Pecchia in the present volume. For the complete hypothetical stemma of the MSS available to the editorial project on *CS Vi* 8, see Philipp A. Maas' paper in the present volume.

[54]This order corresponds to the order of the four epistemological items, excluding *śabda* and beginning with sense perception, that is found in the subsequent text segment characterizing the item *hetu* (see Table 3.4 above); see *CS Vi* 8.33 addressed below, p. 119. It is unanimously confirmed by the manuscript tradition.

22	doubt (*saṃśaya*) (1)
23	motivation (*prayojana*) (2)
24	faltering (?) (*savyabhicāra*) (3)
25	inquisitiveness (*jijñāsā*) (4)
26	determination (*vyavasāya*) (5)

Table 3.8: Terms Denoting Cognitive–Psychological Concepts

aware of the fact that speakers take recourse to different types of knowledge sources in the course of their argumentation.

The epistemological group is followed by a series of terms referring to a range of cognitive–psychological concepts or mental states of participants in a disputation. They may have had to be verbalized and clarified in the context of a disputation (see Table 3.8).

3.1.5.2 Now, according to the *Nyāyabhāṣya* (*NBh*) of Vātsyāyana, some scholars concerned with methodical thinking (*naiyāyikas*)[55] considered five additional elements of argumentation (*avayava*), next to the five elements thesis, etc., assumed in classical Nyāya;[56] these additional elements probably preceded the latter in the resulting scheme of altogether ten elements.[57] Three or even four of the addi-

[55]Oberhammer (1963: 88f.) rightly argues that this term does not specifically refer to followers of a philosophical tradition called Nyāya.

[56]Oetke (1994: 91) considers the lack of these additional elements in the *Nyāyasūtra* a "de-psychologization" of the old Indian syllogism.

[57]See *NBh* 30,8–9 on *NS* 1.1.32. See also *Nyāyamañjarī* (*NM*) II 553,16f. and *Sārasaṅgraha* (*SāS*) 183,7–184,2 on *Tārkikarakṣā* 69 (reference by Mr. Hisataka Ishida, PhD student at the University of Vienna). A variant of this list of ten elements is mentioned by Dharmakīrti's commentator Prajñākaragupta in his commentary on *Pramāṇavārttika* (*PV*) 4.19ab; see Tillemans 1984: 76, n. 9. For a diverging list of ten elements of an argu-

Ten Elements of an Argumentation I (NBh)	*Relevant Topics in* CS Vi *8.27*
inquisitiveness (*jijñāsā*) (1)	inquisitiveness (*jijñāsā*) (4) [25]
doubt (*saṃśaya*) (2)	doubt (*saṃśaya*) (1) [22]
possible attainment [of the aim] (*śakyaprāpti*) (3)	
motivation (*prayojana*) (4)	motivation (*prayojana*) (2) [23]
dispersal of doubt (*saṃśayavyudāsa*) (5)	determination (*vyavasāya*) (5) [26]

Table 3.9: Elements of Argumentation in Nyāya Compared with Relevant Topics in the *Carakasaṃhitā*

tional five elements are obviously related to *pada*s in the present group by direct terminological correspondence and by possible factual identity in spite of terminological differences (see Table 3.9).

In the dialectical tradition of Sāṅkhya as presented in the *Yuktidīpikā* (*YD*) we also encounter these additional *avayavas*.[58] Here they are not simply joined to the well-known five elements, but jointly considered as a *vyākhyāṅga*

mentation in early Jain dialectics, see Ui 1917: 83, with nn. 3 and 4, and Kang 2007: 49.

[58]See *YD* 89,16–18, followed by a long discussion extending up to *YD* 97,5, and the summary in *YD* 4,6–8; see also Frauwallner 1984: 77. Further reference to the ten-fold scheme, without a clear identification of its proponents, is made in Vibhūticandra's notes on the manuscript of the *PV* with Manorathanandin's commentary (reference by Mr. Hisataka Ishida); see the gloss on the first sentence of the commentary on *PV* 4.19ab (p. 420, gloss no. 2). A scheme of additional elements of argumentation termed "expedients" (**aṅga*), starting with inquisitiveness, was also known to Dignāga; see his own commentary on *Pramāṇasam-*

("limb" [i.e., expedient] "of explanation"), preceding the fivefold *pratipādanāṅga* or *parapratyāyanāṅga* ("limb of making [the opponent] understand [one's argument]").[59] The expression *vyākhyāṅga* clearly points at a situation of communication with others and thus verbalization. It should not be overlooked, however, that in the context of the *pada* list of the *Carakasaṃhitā* the group of five terms relating to cognitive–psychological concepts is separated from the relevant group of terms directly relating to the structure of argumentation (nos. 8–13) (see Table 3.4 above), namely, by the group of terms relating to types of statements made at specific stages of a disputation (nos. 14–16) (see Table 3.5 above) and the group of epistemological terms (nos. 17–21) (see Table 3.7 above). Let me add that the present group seems to imply a temporal sequence of its members as regards their relevance and position in the course of the entire process of argumentation right from its inception due to inquisitiveness; however, a sequence extending to and including the five elements that immediately follow within the tenfold scheme reported in the *Nyāyabhāṣya* and the *Yuktidīpikā* can hardly be construed.[60]

3.1.5.3 A similarly diffuse picture, partially matching, partially not matching, results with regard to the group of terms relating to the structure of argumentation in the *pada* list on the one hand (nos. 8–13) (see Table 3.4 above), and the remaining five elements of argumentation in the

uccaya (*PSV*) 4.6 (fol. 65b 6: *des na gźan gyi śes par 'dod pa la sogs pa'i yan lag* ...), referred to already in Tucci 1930: 45, n. 81.

[59]See also Frauwallner 1984: 77; Oberhammer 1963: 96.

[60]For an extensive critical discussion of the ten elements, their functions and relations, including the descriptive and exemplificatory text segments of all involved items in *CS Vi* 8 and the *Nyāyasūtra*, see Kang 2007: 16–49.

larger scheme of ten elements according to the *naiyāyika*s and the fivefold "limb of making the opponent understand one's argument" (*pratipādanāṅga*) according to the Sāṅkhya scheme presented in the *Yuktidīpikā* on the other hand: the five elements of argumentation according to the *Nyāyasūtra*[61] clearly correspond to the five remaining elements of the *naiyāyika*s, and there is a close similarity to the relevant Sāṅkhya set of terms.[62] However, from the point of view of the tenfold as well as the fivefold scheme the element *udāharaṇa* is missing in the pertinent *pada* group (see Table 3.10).

The element *udāharaṇa* may have its factual correspondence in the already mentioned *pada* "generally acknowledged matters" (*dṛṣṭānta*) which figures in the subsequent group of the three *pada*s "replies" (*uttara*), *dṛṣṭānta* and "fixed positions" (*siddhānta*) (nos. 14–16) (see Table 3.5

[61]See the enumeration in *NS* 1.1.32 and the following *sūtras* (33–41) on the individual elements.

[62]The five elements are explicated as elements of the statement of a direct reason (*vītahetu*) in Vārṣagaṇya's *Ṣaṣṭitantra*, to which the author of the *Yuktidīpikā* most probably refers in this context even though the additional five elements may not have been part of Vārṣagaṇya's scheme (see the remarks in *YD* 5,4–8, also referred to and analyzed in Oberhammer 1963: 95f., where it is stated that Vindhyavāsin, who was a disciple and commentator of Vārṣagaṇya, and other masters taught the elements of argumentation starting with inquisitiveness which are jointly called "limb" (i.e., expedient) "of inference" [*anumānāṅga*] in this context). See also Siṃhasūri's *Nyāyāgamānusāriṇī* (*NĀA*) 313, 8–6 and Jinendrabuddhi's *Pramāṇasamuccayaṭīkā*, quoted and analyzed towards the reconstruction of the relevant passage in the *Ṣaṣṭitantra*, in Frauwallner 1958: 88–94 (translation p. 128 f.).

[63]It can be presumed that the terminology of the *naiyāyika*s for the remaining five elements of argumentation making up the set of ten elements was the same as the terminology for the five elements of argumentation in the *Nyāyasūtra*, because Vātsyāyana does not mention any discrepancy in this regard.

[64]See n. 62 for the fivefold scheme probably held by Vārṣagaṇya.

Nyāya (*NS*) (5)	*naiyāyikas* (*NBh*) (10)[63]	Sāṅkhya (5)[64] / (10)	*padas* (*CS Vi* 8.27) (nos. 8–13)
pratijñā (1)	*pratijñā* (6)	*pratijñā* (1) / (6)	*pratijñā* (1) [8] *sthāpanā* (2) [9] *pratiṣṭhāpanā* (3) [10]
hetu (2)	*hetu* (7)	*hetu* (2) / (7)	*hetu* (4) [11]
udāharaṇa (3)	*udāharaṇa* (8)	*dṛṣṭānta* (3) / (8)	
upanaya (4)	*upanaya* (9)	*upasaṃhāra* (4) / (9)	*upanaya* (5) [12]
nigamana (5)	*nigamana* (10)	*nigamana* (5) / (10)	*nigamana* (6) [13]

Table 3.10: Elements of Argumentation

above) which I consider to be a sub-group of the larger group of terms relating to the structure of argumentation and characterized as referring to types of essential statements that have a structurally determined place in a disputation.

Such a rough correspondence in meaning, even though not necessarily in function and structural position within a disputation, is suggested by the fact that the subsequent characterization of *dṛṣṭānta* in the *Carakasaṃhitā* (*Vi* 8.34) is very similar to the characterization of the *padārtha dṛṣṭānta* in the *Nyāyasūtra*:

> What one calls a generally acknowledged matter is something with regard to which the understanding of simple-minded persons and *savants* is the same [and] which describes what is

to be described.[65]

NS 1.1.25 reads:

> A generally acknowledged matter is something with regard to which the understanding of normal people and those who thoroughly examine is the same.[66]

In the order of the sixteen items listed in *NS* 1.1.1[67] and later called *padārtha* in the Nyāya tradition, *dṛṣṭānta* appears rather early among the dialectical terms (no. 5); together with doubt (*saṃśaya*) (no. 3), motivation (*prayojana*) (no. 4) and fixed positions or presuppositions (*siddhānta*) (no. 6) it forms the group immediately preceding the term denoting the five elements of argumentation (*avayava*) (no. 7). According to the respective section title of the division of the *Nyāyasūtra* into sections technically called *prakaraṇa*s, a division which is of uncertain date but certainly postdates Vātsyāyana, the three items *saṃśaya, prayojana* and *dṛṣṭānta* are called "*anterior* limbs of methodical thinking / coherent logical argumentation" (*nyāyapūrvāṅga*); the title of the section treating the five elements of argumentation refers to these elements collectively as the "characterization

---

[65]See *CS Vi* 8.36 (crit. ed.): *dṛṣṭānto nāma yatra mūrkhaviduṣāṃ buddhisāmyam, yo varṇyaṃ varṇayati.* [...]

[66]See *NS* 1.1.25: *laukikaparīkṣakāṇāṃ yasminn arthe buddhisāmyaṃ sa dṛṣṭāntaḥ.* See also the early quotation of the text of this *sūtra* in the introductory comments on **Vaidalyaprakaraṇa* (**VP*) 28 (**VP* p. 33,10f.) and the reference in the commentary on **VP* 9 (**VP* p. 25,3–8, translation p. 62); on the latter passage, see Pind 2001: 161f. (relating to section no. 8, following Kajiyama's enumeration; see Pind's n. 2, p. 149). On the function of *dṛṣṭānta* as characterized in *NS* 1.1.25 and *CS Vi* 8.36 see Oetke 1994: 71f.; for a different interpretation see Oberhammer 1963: 74. See also Frauwallner 1984: 75 and Prets 2004: 200.

[67]See n. 41 above.

of methodical thinking/coherent logical argumentation" (*nyāyalakṣaṇa*). The term *nyāyāṅga* appears already in the *Nyāyavārttika* (*NV*): Uddyotakara affirms in a discussion with other dialecticians that the purpose (*prayojana*) is indeed a "limb of methodical thinking" and thus also of relevance to the right procedure of thorough examination (*parīkṣāvidhi*): no consideration that lacks a purpose can be a "limb of methodical thinking," and the purpose is even a major limb of the right procedure of thorough examination because it is its root.[68] Fixed positions or presuppositions (*siddhānta*), for their part, are the basis of methodical thinking/coherent logical argumentation (*nyāyāśraya*) according to the *prakaraṇa* title (see Table 3.11).

The position of generally acknowledged matters (*dṛṣṭānta*) in the structure of the argumentation – and maybe also their function – is thus a different one according to the *Nyāyasūtra* (and presumably the *naiyāyikas*) and the *vāda* section of the *Carakasaṃhitā*. In the *Nyāyasūtra*, the concept of *dṛṣṭānta* is explicitly integrated into the five elements of argumentation inasmuch as exemplification (*udāharaṇa*) is said to be a generally acknowledged matter (*dṛṣṭānta*) that is characterized by the existence of the relevant property of the thing to be proved (*sādhya*) (i.e., by the existence of its property that is to be proved) because of its similarity with the thing to be proved (i.e., because it undoubtedly possesses also further properties that are similar to / common with properties of the thing to be proved, beyond the property adduced in the proof).[69] Exemplification also figures

[68]See *NV* 97, 4–6 on *NS* 1.1.24: *yad api prayojanaṃ nyāyasyāṅgaṃ na bhavatīti* (see the opponent in *NV* 96, 18f.: *na cānena* [scil. *prayojanena*] *kiñcit parīkṣāvidheḥ kriyata iti nyāyāṅgabhāvo nāstīti*) *tad api na yuktam. yā khalu niṣprayojanā cintā nāsau nyāyasyāṅgam iti. parīkṣāvidhes tu pradhānāṅgaṃ prayojanam eva tanmūlatvāt parīkṣāvidher iti.*

[69]See *NS* 1.1.36: *sādhyasādharmyāt taddharmabhāvī dṛṣṭānta udāharaṇam.*

means of knowledge (*pramāṇa*) (1)	
prameya ([soteriologically relevant] objects of valid cognition) (2)	
doubt (*saṃśaya*) (3) motivation (*prayojana*) (4) generally acknowledged matters (*dṛṣṭānta*) (5)	anterior limbs of methodical thinking (*nyāyapūrvāṅgas*)
fixed positions / presuppositions (*siddhānta*) (6)	basis of methodical thinking (*nyāyāśraya*)
elements of argumentation (*avayava*) (7)	characterization of methodical thinking (*nyāyalakṣaṇa*)

Table 3.11: Items 1–7 in the List of *padārthas* (*Nyāyasūtra* 1.1.1)

in the characterization of the statement of proof or demonstration, the second element of an argumentation according to the *Nyāyasūtra*.[70] In the Sāṅkhya scheme, however, the term *dṛṣṭānta* is used by itself to designate the exemplification in the course of an argumentation[71] (see Table 3.10 above).

[70]See *NS* 1.1.34: *udāharaṇasādharmyāt sādhyasādhanaṃ hetuḥ*.

[71]In *YD* 90,21 (*udāharaṇaṃ tu tannidarśanaṃ dṛṣṭāntaḥ; tat-* refers to *sādhanasya sādhyena sahabhāvitvam*, see *YD* 90,18 and the following explanation), the initial phrase *udāharaṇaṃ tu* is probably an interpolation (see *YD* 93,2 and *NĀA* 314,5) to clarify that function and position of a *dṛṣṭānta* are identical with those of the element of argumentation *udāharaṇa* according to the Nyāya scheme. Similarly, in *YD* 91,4, *upanaya* may have been secondarily added to the characterization of *upasaṃhāra* (see *NĀA* loc. cit.), even though later on in the discussion of the altogether ten items and their characterizations, the term *upanaya* may have replaced the typical *upasaṃhāra* several times already in the original text of the

3.1.5.4 Furthermore, also the other three members of the group of four items preceding the elements of argumentation in the enumeration of the *Nyāyasūtra* (nos. 3, 4 and 6) (see Table 3.11 above) have their terminological correspondences in the *pada* list of the *Carakasaṃhitā*. *siddhānta* (no. 6) occurs right after *dṛṣṭānta* in the former enumeration, like in the *pada* list; however, in the latter the pair appears in this sequence in the second sub-group among the altogether nine terms relating to the structure of argumentation and types of statements in a disputation (see Table 3.5 above), *after* the first sub-group of such terms that comprises the sequential elements of an argumentation starting with the thesis (see Table 3.4 above). Thus, the occurrence of the term *siddhānta* raises similar issues to be discussed as does the term *dṛṣṭānta*, concerning its relative position and precise function in a disputation. And like in the case of the term *dṛṣṭānta*, the respective meanings of the term are nevertheless clearly related; in this case, we even find an identical sub-division into four types of *siddhānta* in the *Nyāyasūtra*[72] and the text segment explaining this topic in the *Carakasaṃhitā*.[73]

saṃśaya and *prayojana* in the list of *NS* 1.1.1 (nos. 3 and 4), the first two "anterior limbs of methodical thinking / coherent logical argumentation" (see Table 3.11 above), on

---

Yuktidīpikā. On *upasaṃhāra* in the syllogism according to the *Ṣaṣṭitantra* see Oetke 1994: 45, n. 31.

On the function and place of the item *dṛṣṭānta* in the context of the forty-four *padas* and other relevant early sources, and on its relation to *udāharaṇa*, see the extensive discussion in Kang 2007: 87–143.

[72]See *NS* 1.1.27: *sa* (scil. *siddhāntaḥ*) *caturvidhaḥ sarvatantrapratitantrādhikaraṇābhyupagamasaṃsthityarthāntarabhāvāt*.

[73]See *CS Vi* 8.37 (crit. ed.): [...] *sa* (scil. *siddhāntaḥ*) *coktaś caturvidhaḥ: sarvatantrasiddhāntaḥ pratitantrasiddhānto 'dhikaraṇasiddhānto 'bhyupagamasiddhānta iti* [...]. See also Frauwallner 1984: 72f.

means of knowledge (*pramāṇa*) (1)	
prameya ([soteriologically relevant] objects of valid cognition (2)	
doubt (*saṃśaya*) (3) motivation (*prayojana*) (4) generally acknowledged matters (*dṛṣṭānta*) (5)	anterior limbs of methodical thinking (*nyāyapūrvāṅgas*)
fixed positions / presuppositions (*siddhānta*) (6)	basis of methodical thinking (*nyāyāśraya*)
elements of argumentation (*avayava*) (7)	characterization of methodical thinking (*nyāyalakṣaṇa*)
reasoning (*tarka*) (8)	
decision (*nirṇaya*) (9)	

Table 3.12: Items 1–9 in the List of *padārthas* (*Nyāyasūtra* 1.1.1)

the other hand, correlate, in this order, with the first two of the *Carakasaṃhitā's* five cognitive–psychological concepts or mental states of participants in a disputation (nos. 22 and 23) from which group of items the present discussion originated (see Table 3.8 above). And – just a reminder – they also appear, although separated by one item, among the first five items of the ten-membered scheme of elements of argumentation of the *naiyāyikas* (nos. 2 and 4, see Table 3.9 above) and are thus also part of the fivefold "limb of explanation" (*vyākhyāṅga*) of certain Sāṅkhya dialecticians (see p. 84 above). Among these five items, we find, as the final item (no. 5), the dispersal of doubt (*saṃśayavyudāsa*); would it therefore be legitimate to suppose that its equivalent in the group of five mental states of participants in a disputation according to the *Carakasaṃhitā* is the final item (no. 5), namely, "determination" (*vyavasāya*) (no. 26 in the *pada* list)[74] (see again Table 3.8 above)? And what about the possibly corresponding Nyāya *padārtha*? Could it be the item "decision" (*nirṇaya*), although in the list of *NS* 1.1.1 this point appears much later in the order of items, as no. 9 *after* the elements of argumentation (*avayava*) (no. 7) and reasoning (*tarka*) as an important method of reflection (no. 8) (see Table 3.12)?

3.1.5.5 From a consideration of the group of five cognitive-psychological concepts or mental states of participants in a disputation in the *pada* list of the *Carakasaṃhitā* (Table 3.8), we have thus moved on to the first five elements of argumentation according to some *naiyāyikas* or the fivefold "limb of explanation" of the Sāṅkhyas (Table 3.9), and further to the remaining five elements of argumentation in the larger scheme of ten elements according to these *naiyāyikas*, the fivefold "limb of making the opponent understand one's position" according to certain Sāṅkhya dialecticians, the five-membered argumentational scheme of the *Nyāyasūtra* and back to the first sub-group of terms relating to the structure of argumentation in the *pada* list of the *vāda* section of the *Carakasaṃhitā* (Table 3.10). From there we revisited the second sub-group of these terms, which may refer to types of essential statements in a disputation (see Table 3.5 above), and from there proceeded to the group of dialectical items immediately *preceding* the (five) elements of argumentation in the *Nyāyasūtra* (Table 3.11) which led us back to the five cognitive–psychological concepts or mental states of participants in a disputation according to

74See Oberhammer 1963: 90.

27	obtainment of the matter (*arthaprāpti*) (1)
28	compatibility/possibility (*sambhava*) (2)
29	something that is open to critical questioning (*anuyojya*) (3)
30	something that is not open to critical questioning (*ananuyojya*) (4)
31	critical questioning (*anuyoga*) (5)
32	critical counter-questioning (*pratyanuyoga*) (6)

Table 3.13: Terms Concerning the Verity of Statements and Their Contents

the *Carakasaṃhitā* (see again Table 3.8), from which we returned to the list of dialectical items in the *Nyāyasūtra*, this time to an item *following* upon the elements of argumentation (Table 3.12). And, as initially stressed, this is not at all an exhaustive treatment because the individual characterizations and exemplifications in *CS Vi* 28–65 were hardly touched upon and further sources remained largely untapped. However, before we might get lost in this maze of probable and possible relationships, correspondences, affinities and transpositions of items in the two major sources for our knowledge of early Indian dialectics upon which I have focussed here, I want to return to the *pada* list of the *vāda* section in the *Carakasaṃhitā*, refraining from further extensive comments on the remaining items and their possible interrelatedness with the Nyāya *padārtha*s.

3.1.6 What seems to provide coherence to the difficult-to-grasp terms of the next group in the list of *pada*s is the fact that they somehow concern the verity of statements uttered in a disputation and of their contents. They are *arthaprāpti*, the obtainment of the matter from another or some other facts, and *sambhava*, the compatibility, appropriateness or

33	faults of speech (*vākyadoṣa*) (1)
34	excellence of speech (*vākyapraśaṃsā*) (2)
35	distortion (*chala*) (3)

Table 3.14: The Forty-four Topics (*CS Vi* 8.27) III – Rhetorical Terms

conformity of a thing, or its possibility;[75] in both cases a certain degree of truth of the matter under discussion may be reasonably assumed. *anuyojya* is something that may be critically questioned, *ananuyojya* its negative counterpart. The perceived degree of verity of statements and their contents is reflected in possible reactions to them; thus, according to the criterion of authorial association suggested by me for this group, the next items, critical questioning and counter-questioning (*anuyoga, pratyanuyoga*), would follow cohesively (see Table 3.13).

3.1.7 From here the list proceeds to rhetorics, again not without coherence, which is provided by the general connection of the last four items of the previous group to this sub-field or side-field of dialectics and eristics. The first two *padas* connected with rhetorics are the items called "faults of speech" (*vākyadoṣa*) and "excellence of speech" (*vākyapraśaṃsā*), to which one can add the next item, namely distortion (*chala*), which relates to the clever twisting and misrepresentation of one's opponent's statements (see Table 3.14).

A larger group of eight further terms centres around the issue of mistakes one may commit in the course of a disputation or charges one may become exposed to, and the subsequent manoeuvres as reactions to them. The list

[75]More on these two topics may be found in 3.5.2.

36 non-demonstrations / non-proofs (*ahetu*) (1)
37 [statements] for which the appropriate time has passed / been transgressed (*atītakāla*) (2)
38 censure (*upālambha*) (3)
39 avoidance / shunning [censure] (*parihāra*) (4)
40 abandoning one's thesis (*pratijñāhāni*) (5)
42 acknowledgement/recognition (*abhyanujñā*) (6)
42 different/further demonstrations/proofs (*hetvantara*) (7)
43 different/further matters (*arthāntara*) (8)
44 points of defeat (*nigrahasthāna*)

Table 3.15: The Forty-four Topics (*CS Vi* 8.27) IV – Terms Relating to Mistakes in a Disputation and Situations Decisive for Final Defeat

is appropriately concluded with *nigrahasthāna*, a term that refers to situations in which one of the participants in the disputation can be stopped from further argumentation[76] and which thus amount to his final defeat (see Table 3.15).

3.1.8 The above brief analytical survey should have made apparent the interface between debate and early philosophical thinking, more precisely, between the serious inquiry into the principles of debate, on the one hand, and the development of epistemology, notably logic, on the other. As indicated above (see p. 79), another "pillar" of philosophy, namely, ontology – not considered to be a characteristic of philosophy by Scharfstein – also has its place in the list of topics relevant to disputation. However, even though ontological basics in the form of six concrete ontological terms appear very early in the *pada* list (nos. 2–7, see Table 3.3 above), they are probably assigned to this

[76]For this interpretation of the term, see Filliozat 1968: 443.

prominent position because of their methodological priority within debate,[77] not because of their priority as regards the traditional and principal interests of the scholars who systematized and theorized the institution and practice of debate.[78] Therefore, this aspect will be passed over in the present context, for the sake of emphasis on the first "pillar" of philosophy, namely, epistemology which includes logic as a characteristic of philosophy.

Reflection on the criteria of a sound demonstration or statement of proof (*hetu*) must have first occurred in connection with this essential step in the formulation of one's own reasoning vis-à-vis an opponent in a disputation (see Table 3.4 above). Similar considerations must have taken place in connection with the identification of *flawed* argumentations: two of the terms concerning mistakes one may commit in a disputation (see Table 3.15 above) explicitly address the demonstration, statement of proof or reason, namely, the term "non-demonstration/non-proof" (*ahetu*) (no. 1; no. 36 in the *pada* list) – in the subsequent explanation of this topic divided into three types[79] – and the "different/

[77]That is, there has to be an understanding about the ontological presuppositions common to the participants in a debate and thus about the possible range of topics of debate.

[78]According to Vidyabhusana (1921: 27), the six ontological terms were borrowed from early Vaiśeṣika and inserted into the *vādamārga* by Caraka himself. On the six Vaiśeṣika categories and their "relatives" in the *Carakasaṃhitā* see especially *Sūtrasthāna* (*Sū*) 1.28f. and 44–52. For a rather detailed exposition see CS[SGAS]: 466–69 and the critical discussion in Narain 1976: 106–10, for a survey of the most important secondary literature on this topic, Comba 1987: 42; see also Meulenbeld 1999: IA, 10 f., with a summary of Comba's discussion of Surendranath Dasgupta's position (Dasgupta 1922) in Comba 1990, which focuses on the concepts of *sāmānya* and *viśeṣa*, and with further references.

[79]See *CS Vi* 8.57: *prakaraṇasama, saṃśayasama, varṇyasama.* On *CS Vi* 8.57 and the problem of the precise meaning of the term *ahetu* see further Kang 2009: 86–91.

further demonstration/proof" (*hetvantara*) (no. 7; no. 42 in the *pada* list), that is, a modified or distorted or, possibly, an additional or accessory proof[80] which may have been impermissibly adduced on top of the proof already stated but not yet substantiated.[81] These are two contexts from which the conceptualization of a logical reason (*hetu*) and its counterpart, the fallacious reason (*hetvābhāsa*) could develop.[82] Another context is naturally that of inference (*anumāna*), one of the five sources of knowledge enumerated in the *pada* list (no. 5; no. 21 in the list) (see Table 3.7 above). Regarding this larger and primarily epistemological context, as opposed to the dialectical–eristic context of theoretical reflections on the proof provided in debate, the *Carakasaṃhitā* offers additional evidence of great interest, some of which was already indicated by Vidyabhusana under his second heading, "*parīkṣā* – the standard of examination," formulated by him to characterize another key doctrine of Medhātithi Gautama included by Caraka in Agniveśa's compendium (see p. 72 above). I will thus turn to this issue now.

3.2.1 To convey the relevant doctrine, Vidyabhusana summarizes in a very condensed manner a few text segments of the eleventh chapter of Caraka's *Sūtrasthāna*. Everything

[80] See Filliozat 1968: 443.

[81] According to the explanation in *CS Vi* 8.63, the "different demonstration/statement of proof" is one that relates to a different topic or matter. See *CS Vi* 8.63 (crit. ed.): *hetvantaraṃ nāma prakṛtihetau vācye vikārahetum āha*. Frauwallner (1984: 70), relying on the printed text of the *Carakasaṃhitā* (*hetvantaraṃ nāma prakṛtahetau vācye yad vikṛtahetum āha*), translates the term as "verfehlte Begründung" (proof that fails its purpose/proof beside the mark), which may correspond to Vidyabhusana's "shifting the reason" (see Vidyabhusana 1921: 35).

[82] See the use of the term *hetvābhāsa* in the explanation of censure (*upālambha*) in *CS Vi* 8.59.

in this world is classified there as twofold, namely, existent (*sat*) and inexistent (*asat*). Its examination (*parīkṣā*) is stated to be fourfold; this is followed by short explications and exemplifications.[83] For a better understanding, it may be useful to present the larger context here, which deserves a brief sketch also for the additional reason that it permits a fleeting glimpse of the importance of the *Carakasaṃhitā* for our knowledge of another "pillar" of Indian philosophy in the early classical period, namely, metaphysics.

3.2.2 The larger context[84] is provided by the topic of three human pursuits,[85] the pursuit of life (*prāṇaiṣaṇā*), that is, of adequate living circumstances, undiminished vital force and exhaustion of the full life-span, the pursuit of wealth (*dhanaiṣaṇā*), and the pursuit of the so-called other world (*paralokaiṣaṇā*),[86] that is, purposeful activity in view of a re-

[83]See Vidyabhusana 1921: 28 relating to *CS Sū* 11.17–25 and 32.

[84]See also the cursory exposition in Dasgupta 1922: 405–8 and the structural survey as well as detailed paraphrase and treatment, with consideration of Cakrapāṇidatta's commentary, in Filliozat 1993. Meindersma (1990: 266 f.) also provides a brief analysis of *CS Sū* 11.2–33. His hypothesis and conclusion that the whole section constitutes a "quite separate" treatise on the proof of rebirth (*paralokasiddhi*) inserted here (pp. 266 and 271–73), however, is not convincing because the section is well embedded in the chapter and connects with other sections of the core *sthānas* of the *Carakasaṃhitā* from a terminological, stylistic and conceptual point of view. Roşu rightly characterizes the examination of the "other world" as an exemplary expression of the rational attitude of the Indian medical scientists applied here to substantiate a doctrine that was not developed on rational grounds (1978b: 79); see similarly Filliozat 1990: 34. See n. 99 below on a diametrically opposed Marxist view about this section.

[85]On the derivation and meaning of the word *eṣaṇā* see Filliozat 1993: 94 f.

[86]See *CS Sū* 11.3. The pursuit of life is treated in *CS Sū* 11.4, the pursuit of wealth in 11.5. This triad may be an adaptation of the older concept of three human pursuits (*putreṣaṇā, vitteṣaṇā, lokeṣaṇā*) found in the *Bṛhad-*

newed existence in another setting,[87] especially and foremost a heavenly existence.[88] The exposition of the third pursuit starts from the perennial question "Will we continue to exist after we have passed away from this world, or not?",[89] which throws basic doubt on the existence of the "other world" as a goal of human aspiration. This provides the author with the occasion to mention those who – relying on sense perception only and thus adopting the well-known epistemological position of most Indian materialist philosophers[90] – deny repeated existence (*punarbhava*);[91] he then presents, in a concise verse, different views on the single basic cause of human birth[92] that all amount to a rejection

---

āraṇyaka-Upaniṣad (*BṛU*) (3.5.1 and 4.4.22). See Filliozat 1993: 96 and, though inconclusive, Das 1993: 36–38; Roşu (1978a: 258 f.) speaks of a "résonance upaniṣadique" when he discusses the integration of the three human goals (*trivarga*) into the three human pursuits of *CS Sū* 11.3, which he considers as the basic values of medical philosophy. The continuing importance of the concept of three pursuits is documented by the fact that in a formula employed in the context of undertaking *saṃnyāsa*, the renouncer states that he has "risen from" these three pursuits, i.e., distanced and emancipated himself from them; see, e.g., the two quotations from the *Viśveśvarapaddhati* and Kapila in the early-modern *Yatidharmaprakāśa* (*YP*) (p. 46,1f. and 19f.).

[87]See also Filliozat's remarks on the usage of *paraloka* in the present context (1990: 34). See further Steinkellner 1984: 87 on the term *paraloka* from a historical perspective that can also be applied with slight adjustment to its usage in the non-Buddhist traditions.

[88]For a discussion of the meaning of *paraloka* in the context of *CS Sū* 11.3 in combination with 11.33, see Das 1993: 35 f.

[89]See *bhaviṣyāma itaś cyutā na veti* in *CS Sū* 11.6; the treatment of *paralokaiṣaṇā* continues until *Sū* 11.33.

[90]See also Meindersma 1990: 270 and Meindersma 1992: 301.

[91]See the quotation in n. 95 below.

[92]See *CS Sū* 11.6: *mātaraṃ pitaraṃ caike manyante janmakāraṇam / svabhāvaṃ paranirmāṇaṃ yadṛcchāṃ cāpare janāḥ / /*. On the causes *svabhāva* and *yadṛcchā*, cp. the verse *Śvetāśvatara-Upaniṣad* (*ŚU*) 1.2 which answers, *inter alia*, the question "From what were we born?" (*kutaḥ sma jātāḥ*) (fur-

of repeated existence. In the following, he refutes his first-mentioned opponents' premise, namely, that perception is the only reliable source of knowledge, which allegedly results in the claim that only that which is perceptible exists in this world.[93] Next, the author discusses, rejects and denigrates the different views on the cause of birth.[94] When he sketches the last position – explicitly labelled "heretic" (*nāstika*)[95] – that the cause of human birth is pure chance (*yadṛcchā*), and adduces some denials typical for proponents of this position,[96] he stresses the fact that for this opponent neither examination (*parīkṣā*) nor an object to be examined (*parīkṣya*) exists.[97] Thus, the transition to the fourfold examination of what exists and what does not exist is well prepared, and after a general characterization and exemplification of examination,[98] the author proceeds to apply examination to repeated existence as an object of examina-

---

ther on this famous verse see Oberlies 1995: 79 f., with references). See also *Suśrutasaṃhitā* (*SS*) *Śārīrasthāna* (*Śā*) 1.11f. (referred to in Dasgupta 1922: 372 and 410), which addresses further first causes also mentioned in *ŚU* 1.2.

[93]See *CS Sū* 11.7f. On the causes for the non-perception of existent and in principle perceptible things listed in text segment 8, see Preisendanz 1994: 530–40.

[94]See *CS Sū* 11.9–16.

[95]See also the abstract noun *nāstikya* in the earlier sentence *santi hy eke pratyakṣaparāḥ parokṣatvāt punarbhavasya nāstikyam āśritāḥ* (*CS Sū* 11.6) and in 11.7, and the expression *nāstikagraha* immediately afterwards in 11.15cd (a passage which Chattopadhyaya (1977: 375) considers a demonstration of "abject servility" of the doctors to the "law-givers").

[96]In the context of *CS Sū* 11.14f., the term *nāstika* is described by means of reference to the negation of ideas and concepts that are mainly of relevance in traditional or "orthodox" belief and pertain to ethics and soteriology (see the keywords *kartṛ, kāraṇa, karman* and *karmaphala*) as well as mythology and legendary tradition (see the reference to *devas*, *ṛṣis* and *siddhas*).

[97]See *CS Sū* 11.14a.

[98]See *CS Sū* 11.18–26c.

tion, which – not unexpectedly – turns out to be something which indeed exists.[99]

3.2.3 The general as well as the applied section on "examination" make it evident that *parīkṣā*[100] here refers to various means and modes of examination,[101] rather than to the act of examination as such. The four types of *parīkṣā* are accordingly called "measures" or "means of valid cognition" (*pramāṇa*) in the final text segment on the pursuit of the "other world",[102] where the author proceeds,

---

[99] See *CS Sū* 11.26d-32. On the section starting with the classification of all that exists as *sat* and *asat*, and on the subsequent general treatment of the means of examination, see Dasgupta 1922: 373–77 (with extensive reference to Cakrapāṇidatta's commentary) and 398–401, and Biardeau 1964: 444–46. On the section where examination is applied to repeated existence, see Dasgupta 1922: 406–8.

Chattopadhyaya considers the section *CS Sū* 11.3–33 as an example of a discussion that does not have a legitimate place in a medical work; it is an "alien element" and has "the nature of a ransom offered to the counter-ideology without which it is not easy for the doctors to save their science" from the attacks by orthodox "law-givers," even though this strategy results in the crippling of the science by its opposite; in Chattopadhyaya's Marxist–materialistic perspective, the "concession to the metaphysics of the soul" as evidenced in *CS Sū* 11.3–33 goes "against the fundamentals of medical science" and means "the rejection of the methodology of science," according to which the primary epistemological position belongs to direct perception or empirical knowledge (Chattopadhyaya 1977: 375–78). For a diametrically opposed judgement see below, p. 118.

[100] Literally: "looking all around;" on this etymology see Preisendanz 1994: 693.

[101] Filliozat interprets *parīkṣā* as an "attitude of mind" (1993: 102) and speaks of it as a "faculty" that is "a characteristic of man, which he uses in normal conditions of health" (*ibid.*, p. 110).

[102] See *CS Sū* 11.33: *evaṃ pramāṇaiś caturbhir upadiṣṭe punarbhave* ...; see also Roşu's implicit observation regarding this important terminological issue (1978b: 88) which has been neglected by practically all other scholars concerned with the topic (for an exception, see Filliozat 1990: 34) who speak about the concept and number, etc., of the *pramāṇas* in the

upon the establishment of repeated existence, to admonish his listeners/readers to be attentive with regard to the so-called portals of duty or portals to merit (*dharmadvāra*),[103] which comprise *inter alia* obedience to one's teacher, studying, production of offspring, charity and composition/stabilization (*samādhi*) of the mind, and recommends to them all other activities not disapproved by good people that will eventually provide fame in this world and the attainment of heaven after passing away. Specifically, the four means or modes of examination are the instruction by or tradition of trustworthy persons, sense perception, inference and *yukti*.[104]

Among them, *yukti* is a remarkable source of knowledge which may have been a special, innovative feature of the *Carakasaṃhitā* or a specific part of its tradition[105] and which is only treated here.[106] It was specifically considered and criticized by Śāntarakṣita, the ninth-century Buddhist scholar in his survey of the major metaphysical and epistemological tenets of the classical philosophical tra-

---

Carakasaṃhitā, as if this generic term were well established there. In *CS Vi* 4.4, only the instruction by trustworthy persons (*āptopadeśa*) is explicitly called an "authority" (or "means of knowledge"?) (*pramāṇa*); cf. also the possibly terminological expression *pramāṇīkṛtya* referring to *yukti* (see below) in *Vi* 8.149. Again, tradition (*āgama*) is stated to be a *pramāṇa* in the first chapter of the conceptually rather heterogeneous *Śārīrasthāna* (*Śā* 1.45), where much later on the three knowledge sources perception, inference and instruction are explicitly and jointly designated with this term (see *Śā* 6.28, quoted in n. 138).

[103]This may refer to a specific genre of teachings; see *CS Sū* 11.28. Cp. also the description of trustworthy persons (*āpta*) as *dharmadvārāvahita* in *CS Sū* 11.29.

[104]*CS Sū* 11.17: ...*āptopadeśaḥ pratyakṣam anumānaṃ yuktiś ceti*; in 11.27 the first knowledge source is termed *āptāgama*.

[105]See also Filliozat 1990: 45.

[106]See also Filliozat 1990: 38.

ditions;[107] in verse 1692b of the *Tattvasaṅgraha*, Śāntarakṣita expressly refers to the sage (*muni*) Caraka in this connection.[108] *yukti*, as presented in the context of the pursuit of the "other world," can be characterized as a mode of reasoning which takes into consideration a multiplicity of diverse, but conjoined factors, and their adequacy and coherence vis-à-vis a specific outcome.[109] The well-known four means

[107]See *TS* 1691–1697. Cakrapāṇidatta was well aware of Śāntarakṣita's reference and criticism, as well as of Kamalaśīla's comments on these verses; in his extensive commentary on *CS Sū* 11.25 he quotes *TS* 1691f., 1695 and 1697.

[108]On Śāntarakṣita's exposition and criticism of *yukti* see Dasgupta 1922: 375 f.; see also Filliozat 1993: 109 and especially Filliozat 1990: 39–44, which includes a careful and well-reasoned criticism of Dasgupta's exposition, interpretational approach and final judgement.

[109]See *CS Sū* 11.23–25: *jalakarṣaṇabījartusaṃyogāt sasyasambhavaḥ / yuktiḥ ṣaḍdhātusaṃyogād garbhāṇāṃ sambhavas tathā // mathyamanthakamanthānasaṃyogād agnisambhavaḥ / yuktiyuktā catuṣpādasampad vyādhinibarhaṇī // buddhiḥ paśyati yā bhāvān bahukāraṇayogajān / yuktis trikālā sā jñeyā trivargaḥ sādhyate yayā //*; on these verses, see especially Filliozat 1990: 34–36. See further the examplification of *yukti*, by way of application to the issue of repeated existence, in text segment 32, discussed in Filliozat 1990: 37 and, more extensively, in Filliozat 1993: 108–10: *yuktiś caiṣā – ṣaḍdhātusamudayād garbhajanma, kartṛkaraṇasaṃyogāt kriyā, kṛtasya karmaṇaḥ phalaṃ nākṛtasya, nāṅkurotpattir abījāt, karmasadṛśaṃ phalam, nānyasmād bījād anyasyotpattir iti yuktiḥ* (see also Roşu 1978b: 84). My interpretation of *yukti* is close to that by Pierre-Sylvain Filliozat (see especially his paraphrase in Filliozat 1990: 35) and eventually concurs with Jean Filliozat's sensitive understanding of *yukti* as the attitude of mind of a practising physician, an understanding which is outlined on the basis of oral tradition in Filliozat 1993: 111 and, in more detail, in Filliozat 1990: 44 (see also Filliozat 1968: 441: "le traitement synthétisant de l'information"); Roşu characterizes *yukti* as "l'idée d'un concours de plusieurs élements qui, par ajustement rationnel, aboutissent à une représentation cohérente d'un phénomène (Roşu, loc. cit.; similarly Filliozat 1968: 440 f.), which echoes and synthesizes further translation equivalents, or elements of them, suggested by Filliozat père (see Filliozat 1990: 44). Larson's evaluation of *yukti* as "heuristic reasoning" and as referring to "an empirical and, indeed, experimental scientific (in the modern sense) approach to

of knowledge of classical Nyāya do *not* include *yukti*, but comprise comparison/analogy (*upamāna*) instead, which is also found with a slightly diverging term (*aupamya*) in the group of five epistemological terms in the list of *pada*s (see Table 3.16; see also Table 3.7 above).

Vidyabhusana is therefore uncertain whether the fourfold "standard of examination" as found in *CS Sū* 11 or the corresponding three knowledge sources plus comparison, as found in *CS Vi* 8, represent the epistemology of Medhātithi Gautama as adopted in the *Carakasaṃhitā*.[113]

---

reality and experience" (see Larson 1987: 250 f.), which reminds one of Filliozat's further understanding of *yukti* as referring to the establishment of a theory (Filliozat 1990: 44), also catches some of the "flavour" of *yukti*, even though his treatment of *CS Sū* 11.23–25 is quite unsatisfactory. On other usages of the word *yukti*, which is frequently used in the *Carakasaṃhitā*, in a technical and non-technical sense, see Filliozat 1990: 37 f.; Filliozat rightly stresses that it would be a mistake to look for a single common character of these usages, beyond the broad etymological link, and unify the underlying notions (1990: 45).

For a study of the term *yukti*, with a focus on its employment in Buddhist literature, see Scherrer-Schaub 1981, where reference is made *inter alia* – in reliance on Biardeau's treatment (see n. 99 above) – to the means of investigation called *yukti* in *CS Sū* 11 (p. 192). On the different types of *yukti* or "reasoning" in the *Abhidharmasamuccaya* and its commentary (*ASBh*), see Prets 1994: 343–45, on the classification and types of *yukti* according to the *Sandhinirmocanasūtra* and other early Yogācāra treatises, including the *Abhidharmasamuccaya*, see Yoshimizu 1996 (with an English summary on pp. 160–64) and Yoshimizu 2010: 140, n. 2; Yoshimizu 2010 is devoted to the so-called *upapattisādhanayukti*. On *yukti* in Dharmaśāstra, see Preisendanz 2010: 55, with nn. 101f. (with further references).

[110]*pramāṇa*s according to *Sū* 11.33; see n. 102 above.

[111]*NS* 1.1.3 reads: *pratyakṣānumānopamānaśabdāḥ pramāṇāni*.

[112]On the sequence of these *pada*s adopted here, see p. 82 above.

[113]See Vidyabhusana 1921: 27. As Vidyabhusana himself is doubtful whether the doctrine he summarizes under his first heading ("the aggregate of resources for the accomplishment of an action") (see p. 72 above) is at all to be connected with Medhātithi Gautama's "investig-

CS Sū 11.17 (*parīkṣās*)[110]	*NS* 1.1.3 (*pramāṇas*)[111]	*CS Vi* 8.27 (*padas* 17–21)[112]
instruction by trustworthy persons (*āptopadeśa*)	sense perception (*pratyakṣa*)	verbal testimony (*śabda*)
sense perception (*pratyakṣa*)	inference (*anumāna*)	sense perception (*pratyakṣa*)
inference (*anumāna*)	comparison/analogy (*upamāna*)	comparison/analogy (*aupamya*)
yukti	verbal testimony (*śabda*)	oral tradition (*aitihya*)
		inference (*anumāna*)

Table 3.16: Epistemological Items

3.2.4 A word is due here on the term *śabda*. When Vidyabhusana briefly treats the above two relevant passages of the *Carakasaṃhitā* on the sources of knowledge in his *History*, he clearly understands *śabda* (literally: "word") in the *pada* list (*Vi* 8.27) in the sense of verbal testimony, equating it with instruction by trustworthy persons (*āptopadeśa*) in the *paralokaiṣaṇā* section (*Sū* 11.17), and does not refer to *aitihya* ("oral tradition"), which occurs in penultimate position in the relevant group of five epistemological terms in the *pada* list.[114] A little later, however, in the context of his brief exposition of the forty-four *padas*, he renders

ating [science]" (see Vidyabhusana loc. cit.), there is no need to enter into it here.

[114]See Vidyabhusana 1921: 27.

śabda with "word",[115] explained by him as "a combination of letters." Vidyabhusana consequently understands *aitihya* to refer to a fourth (and not fifth) means of knowledge here, in addition to sense perception, inference and comparison/analogy,[116] which is to be equated with *āptopadeśa* in the *paralokaiṣaṇā* section of *Sū* 11.[117] The listing of the term "word," however, would be contextually inappropriate here and Vidyabhusana's interpretation as well as his explanation of the term as referring to "a combination of letters" seems to be based on a misunderstanding of the subsequent explanation of the term *śabda* in the *vāda* section itself.[118] Furthermore, the harmonization and mutual

---

[115]See Vidyabhusana 1921: 33 (followed, e.g., by Hedge 1976: 18, Solomon 1976: 80 and Sharma 1994: 362). See also, e.g., Filliozat 1968: 442 ("parole") and Sharma and Dash 1994: 232 ("words").

[116]Thus the order adopted by Vidyabhusana. I could not yet clarify on which edition of the *Carakasaṃhitā* Vidyabhusana based his research. However, this order is found in three early editions published in Kolkata accessible to the projects mentioned in the acknowledgement note on p. 63 above, namely, the second edition of Jivananda Vidyasagara Bhattacaryya's edition (Narayan Press 1896), and the editions with translations into Bengali by Avinash Chandra Kaviratna Kaviraj (Vidyaratna Press 1884/1885) and Yashodanandan Sarkar (second edition; Vangavasi Electro Machine Press 1910/1911). It is less probable that Vidyabhusana relied on the edition, with Marathi translation and notes, by Shankar Daji Shastri Pade (Mumbai: Yajneshvar Gopal Dikshit, Bookseller 1897–1898, with three further editions printed by various presses in Mumbai and Pune during 1901 and 1914).

[117]See similarly Filliozat 1968: 442.

[118]See *CS Vi* 8.38 (crit. ed.): *śabdo nāma varṇasamāmnāyaḥ. sa dṛṣṭārthaś cādṛṣṭārthaś ca satyaś cānṛtaś ceti. tatra dṛṣṭārthaḥ: tribhir hetubhir doṣāḥ prakupyanti, ṣaḍbhir upakramaiś ca praśāmyanti, śrotrādisadbhāve śabdādigrahaṇam iti. adṛṣṭārthaḥ punaḥ: asti pretyabhāvaḥ, asti mokṣa iti. satyaḥ satyo nāma: santy āyurvedopadeśāḥ, santy upāyāḥ sādhyānām, santy ārambhaphalānīti. satyaviparyayāc cānṛtaḥ.* In this explanation, I understand the term *varṇasamāmnāya* as meaning "the collocation of [articulate] sounds" (see Böhtlingk 1883–1886: s.v. *samāmnāya*, 1) … "Zusammenstellung"); such a col-

adjustment of the two passages attempted by Vidyabhusana in this way is, in my view, not necessary, or even unjustified, if one generally acknowledges the possibility of additions to the core text of the *Carakasaṃhitā* and specifically assumes that the *vāda* section is an interpolation in *CS Vi* 8 (see above, 3.1.2).

Even so, it is necessary to reflect on the precise difference between *śabda* (no. 17) and *aitihya* (no. 20)[119] in the *pada* list. It may well be that in the first case an author or individual agent of the statement is involved, i.e., a concrete speaker who is the source or transmitter of the verbally conveyed knowledge, whereas in the second case the list refers to oral tradition, i.e., statements of a less personal nature and authority, such as the statements constituting the Vedic corpus proclaimed by superhuman speakers.[120] This would amount to a categorical distinction between

---

location, i.e., a statement, may be true, but also untrue, namely, in the case of erroneous personal statements and statements based on unaccepted, unauthoritative rival traditions. It seems that the explanation adduced here stems from another context where human statements as such are classified, and not human statements as a means of knowledge relevant in debate, because in this latter context it would be redundant to characterize one type as true (*satya*) – a source of knowledge is true by definition –, whereas the characterization of its diametrically opposed type as untrue (*anṛta*) would be out of place. For another case of a discrepant explication of a term in the *pada* list, see, e.g., the explication of the term *hetu* referred to in n. 54 above and addressed on p. 119 below. As already indicated by Frauwallner (1984: 70, n. 16), the explanations of the individual *padas* should not necessarily be considered as originally linked to the *padas* in the list; they are thus not necessarily authoritative as regards the interpretation of the listed terms.
On the misunderstanding of *varṇa* as referring to a letter, see Wezler 1994.

[119]On the sequential number of this *pada* see above, p. 82.

[120]See the subsequent explanation in *CS Vi* 8.41 (crit. ed.) (on this segment numbering see again above, p. 82): *aitihyaṃ nāmāptopadeśo vedādiḥ*.

individual reliable human statements, perhaps including also tradition-based statements, and the authoritative tradition of legendary or mythical speakers as two separate sources of knowledge.[121] As is well known, according to the *Nyāyasūtra* these are the two types of the means of knowledge that is there called "verbal testimony" (*śabda*). Intriguingly, in their respective characterization as "having a seen object/content" (*dṛṣṭārtha*), i.e., an object/content that is accessible in this world by way of normal human experience, and "having an unseen object/content" (*a-dṛṣṭārtha*), i.e., an object/content that is inaccessible in this way,[122] we re-encounter the terms used to designate the first two types of verbal testimony, or more precisely, of human statements as such, in the explanation of the term *śabda* in the *vāda* section of *CS Vi* 8.[123] Furthermore, the verbal testimony of the *Nyāyasūtra* is basically characterized as "instruction by trustworthy persons" (*āptopadeśa*), which is the designation of the first means of examination (*parīkṣā*) according to *CS Sū* 11.17. According to Vātsyāyana, these trustworthy persons (*āpta*s) may be ordinary human beings *and* seers,[124] something which may also be implied in the characterization of *āptopadeśa*, under the heading *āptāgama* ("tradition of trustworthy persons"), in *CS Sū* 11.27, when this means of examination is applied to the problem of repeated birth, even though in this text segment the involved group of ordinary human beings

---

[121]See also Frauwallner 1984: 70: "Mitteilung" and "Überlieferung."

[122]See *NS* 1.1.7f.: *āptopadeśaḥ śabdaḥ. sa dvividho dṛṣṭādṛṣṭārthatvāt.*

[123]See *CS Vi* 8.38, quoted above, n. 118.

[124]See *NBh* 14,10f. on *NS* 1.1.8: *yasya* (scil. *śabdasya*) *iha dṛśyate 'rthaḥ sa dṛṣṭārthaḥ. yasyāmutra pratīyate so 'dṛṣṭārthaḥ. evam ṛṣilaukikavākyānāṃ vibhāga iti.*

is limited to *savants*.[125] Such a dual division of agents of instruction, however, does not occur in the general characterization of trustworthy persons provided – instead of a characterization of *āptopadeśa* – in *CS Sū* 11.18f.[126] *aitihya*, for its part, figures as the first item in the brief discussion and rejection of possible further means of knowledge, beyond the four accepted in Nyāya, at the beginning of the second *adhyāya* of the *Nyāyasūtra* (*NS* 2.2.1f.); there, *aitihya* is not considered an additional source of knowledge because it is nothing but verbal testimony (*śabda*) according to the Nyāya understanding.[127] The same argumentation can be found in some classical Sāṅkhya sources, foremost among them the *Yuktidīpikā*.[128]

The terminological relationship between the three main

---

[125]See *CS Sū* 11.27: *tatrāptāgamas tāvad vedaḥ. yaś cānyo 'pi vedārthād aviparītaḥ parīkṣakaiḥ praṇītaḥ śiṣṭānumato lokānugrahapravṛttaḥ śāstravādaḥ sa cāptāgamaḥ.* [...] On this text segment see, e.g., Biardeau 1964: 445, Filliozat 1968: 441, Hedge 1976: 19, Chattopadhyaya 1977: 377, Roşu 1978b: 92 f. and Filliozat 1993: 102 f. In the difficult characterization of trustworthy persons in the clinical context of diagnosis in *CS Vi* 4 (see below, p. 115), the term seems to be even further restricted to saintly persons whose knowledge is of a supernormal kind (see *CS Vi* 4.4; see also Filliozat 1968: 441 and Roşu 1978b: 90).

[126]See *CS Sū* 11.18f.: *rajastamobhyāṃ nirmuktās tapojñānabalena ye / yeṣāṃ trikālam amalaṃ jñānam avyāhataṃ sadā // āptāḥ śiṣṭā vibudhās te, teṣāṃ vākyam asaṃśayam / satyam, vakṣyanti te kasmād asatyaṃ nīrajastamāḥ //.* See also, e.g., Hedge 1976: 18 and Roşu 1978b: 90 f. on these verses.

[127]See *NS* 2.2.1f.: *na catuṣṭvam aitihyārthāpattisambhavābhāvaprāmāṇyāt. śabda aitihyānarthāntarabhāvāt ... apratiṣedhaḥ.*

[128]See *YD* 71, 3–6. Ruben (1928: 40) already refers to a parallel verdict in Gauḍapāda's *Bhāṣya* on *Sāṅkhyakārikā* (*SK*) 4 (see *GPBh* 9, 13). See similarly *Jayamaṅgalā* (*JM*) 69, 23f.; for a summary of this position in the short commentaries *Sāṅkhyasaptativṛtti* and *Sāṅkhyavṛtti*, see Solomon 1974: 11 f. In the commentary on the *Sāṅkhyakārikā* translated into Chinese by Paramārtha, *aitihya* is not specifically mentioned, but certainly one among the six possible further sources of knowledge to be included in *āptavacana* ("statement of trustworthy persons" / "trustworthy

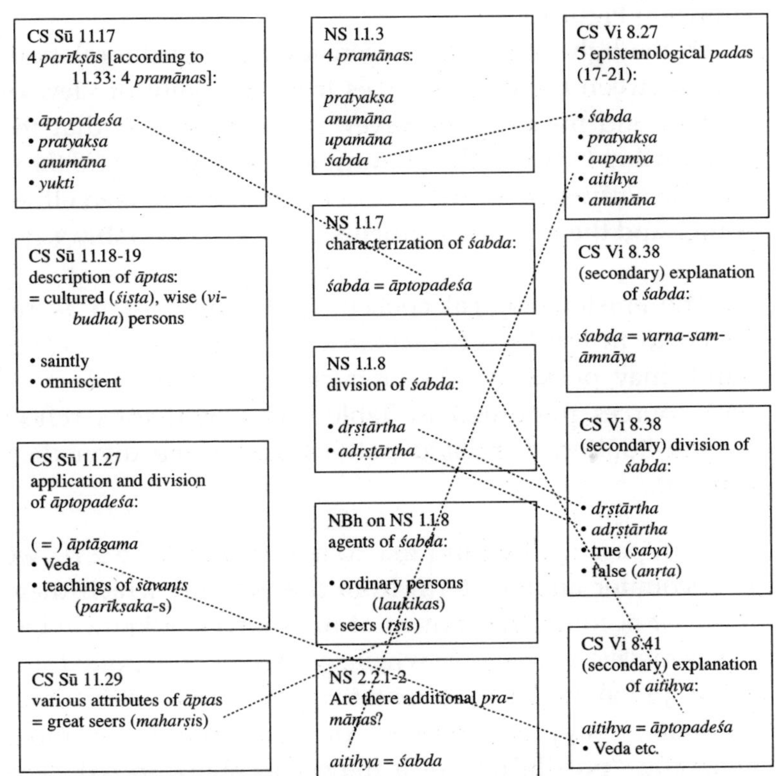

Figure 3.3: The Terminological Criss-Cross Related to "Instruction by Trustworthy Persons" and "Verbal Testimony" in *CS Sū* 11.17–19, 27 and 29, *CS Vi* 8.27,[a] 38 and 41,[b] and the *NS*.

[a]For the order of the *padas*, see above, p. 82.

[b]This numbering follows the order of the explanatory text segments established in the new critical edition of *CS Vi* 8; see above, p. 82.

sources for our knowledge of the relevant means of knowledge which were adduced above may thus be presented as shown in Figure 3.3.

In the light of the above consideration of the relationship between the three sources from the point of view of content and meaning, however, it becomes clear that the relationship between the relevant text segments in *CS Sū* 11 and the *Nyāyasūtra* is much closer than that between either source and the relevant segments in *CS Vi* 8 (see Table 3.17).

The epistemological concept under discussion as referred to in the list of *padas* in *CS Vi* 8.27, on the other hand, may possibly[129] be characterized as in Table 3.18. *Both* sources presented in Table 3.17 would thus reflect a consolidation of related notions under one diversified concept.

3.2.5 In passing, I would like to add that in *NS* 2.2.1f. we re-encounter another term from the *pada* list which there does *not* occur in the context of the sources of knowledge; this is *sambhava*,[130] a term which, guided by the context (see Table 3.13 above), I have tentatively rendered with "compatibility," "appropriateness" or "conformity," or more generally, "possibility," of a thing (see above, p. 94). Literally meaning "being together," this additional means of

statement"), the term employed in *SK* 4 for the means of knowledge under discussion here (see Takakusu 1904: 984).

[129]This uncertainty is due to the doubtful status of the subsequent characterizations and exemplifications of the individual items in the list; see n. 118 above.

[130]Frauwallner (1984: 72), who disregards the internal associative logic that is possibly at the basis of the order of terms in the *pada* list, simply assumes that *sambhava* (as well as the preceding item *arthaprāpti*) is part of a series of terms starting with *śabda* and referring to means of knowledge, even though other terms intervene.

Carakasaṃhitā Sūtrasthāna 11	*Nyāyasūtra*
instruction by/tradition of trustworthy persons (*āptopadeśa, āptāgama*)	verbal testimony (*śabda*)
division into • Veda • teachings by means of / in the form of bodies of expert knowledge (*śāstravāda*)	division into verbal testimony • having an "unseen" object/content (*adṛṣṭārtha*) (2) • having a "seen" object/content (*dṛṣṭārtha*) (1)
agents: • cultured (*śiṣṭa*) and wise (*vibudha*) persons (saintly, omniscient), great seers (*maharṣis*) • *savants* (*parīkṣakas*)	agents (according to the *NBh*): • seers (*ṛṣis*) • ordinary human beings (*laukikas*)

Table 3.17: Relationship Between *Carakasaṃhitā* and *Nyāyasūtra*

knowledge suggested by some opponent(s) in *NS* 2.2.1 is explained differently by Vātsyāyana in his commentary on this *sūtra*, namely, as the grasping of the existence of one thing on account of the grasping of the existence of another thing that is invariably connected with it; the example provided by Vātsyāyana points to the more specific idea of this relationship as inclusion.[131] Furthermore, the term

[131]See *NBh* 99, 10–12: *sambhavo nāmāvinābhāvino 'rthasya sattāgrahaṇād anyasya sattāgrahaṇam. yathā droṇasya sattāgrahaṇād āḍhakasya sattāgraha-*

śabda (no. 17)	*aitihya* (no. 20)
personal communication	oral tradition
individual human speakers	legendary / mythical speakers

Table 3.18: *CS Vi* 8.27: Epistemological Concepts

referring to the possible additional means of knowledge mentioned just before *sambhava* in *NS* 2.2.1, implication or circumstantial evidence (*arthāpatti*), a well-known typical feature of Mīmāṃsā epistemology, is reminiscent of the term *arthaprāpti* ("obtainment [of the matter] from [another / some other] fact(s)"), which also precedes *sambhava* as a *pada* in *CS Vi* 8.27, in the context of the terms concerning the verity of statements uttered in a disputation and of their contents (see again Table 3.13); depending on whether one assumes a transitive or intransitive meaning of the word *prāpti* ("obtainment"), *arthaprāpti* may be understood more precisely as the intellectual attainment or following of one thing from another / some other fact(s).[132]

3.2.6 Let me return to the means of knowledge referred to in the *Carakasaṃhitā*. As we have seen, there are two

ṇam āḍhakasya grahaṇāt prasthasyeti. On this characterization see also, e.g., Solomon 1976: 451. For further references to various characterizations, descriptions and illustrations of *sambhava* found in the classical literature, inclusive of the medical tradition, see Oberhammer *et al.* 2006: s.v. *sambhava*.

[132] Oberhammer (1991: s.v. *arthaprāpti*) assumes that "judging from the linguistic form" (?) ("der sprachlichen Form nach") *arthaprāpti* is an older variant of the term *arthāpatti*. *prāpti* (intransitive) and *āpatti* (and other derivations from the two roots with their respective preverbs, such as *prāpyate* and *āpadyate*), are indeed used synonymously, although I would refrain from construing a historical priority of either one to the other.

different sets of them appearing in two different contexts. Beyond these, means of knowledge figure in the context of diagnostics. One short text segment is found in the part of *CS Vi* 8 following upon the list of forty-four *padas*, in the long excursus that may be entitled "How to act successfully" and concludes this chapter (*CS Vi* 8.68–151; see Table 3.2 above). Before the author proceeds to explain in much detail ten topical complexes (*prakaraṇa*) as items to be examined (*parīkṣya*) by a physician before he begins his treatment, he briefly introduces the means or modes of examination. As in *CS Sū* 11, the relevant expression here is *parīkṣā*. However, the means of examination mentioned in this context are basically just two, sense perception and inference, supplemented by instruction (*upadeśa*).[133] The distinctive means of knowledge called *yukti* is missing here,[134] and instruction by others, even though not completely lacking, takes a back seat in the present context, probably because it is not directly involved in the actual process of diagnostic examination. This interpretation is suggested by a further passage found at the beginning of the fourth chapter of the *Vimānasthāna* which is devoted to the diagnosis of diseases. The term initially used here is *rogaviśeṣavijñāna*, where the word *vijñāna* has to be understood as referring to *means* of in-depth knowledge, not to the process, similar to the special usage of the word *parīkṣā* in *CS Sū* 11 and *Vi* 8.83 (see above, p. 102). These means are three: instruction by trustworthy persons, sense perception

[133]See *CS Vi* 8.83 (crit. ed.): *dvividhā parīkṣā jñānavatām – pratyakṣam anumānaṃ ca. etat tu dvayam upadeśaś ca parīkṣātrayam. evam eṣā dvividhā parīkṣā, trividhā vā sahopadeśena.*

[134]See also Cakrapāṇidatta's remarks about the lack of the item *yukti* in *Vi* 4.5 (see below) and *Vi* 8 (specifically in the *pada* list) and his explanation of this situation in his commentary on *Sū* 11.25 (ĀD 72a, 5–15), already pointed out in Filliozat 1990: 42.

and inference.[135] The order is explained a little later on from the clinical point of view: instruction by trustworthy persons indeed comes first; only thereafter examination (*parīkṣā*) by means of sense perception and inference is possible. For how could a person who examines something by means of sense perception and inference know, i.e., understand, this thing if he has not been instructed on it before?! Therefore the means of examination (*parīkṣā*) is in fact twofold for knowledgeable persons: sense perception and inference, or threefold, together with the preceding instruction.[136] Three subsequent text segments explain and exemplify the acquisition of medical knowledge by means of instruction, sense perception and inference.[137] In the conclusion of the segment on sense perception, the actual order of means of examination established at the end of the explanation from the clinical point of view is confirmed: in spite of the primacy of instruction, in the context of actual, concrete examination sense perception and inference come first.[138] For the context of diagnostics, the concept of means

---

[135]See *CS Vi* 4.3: *trividhaṃ khalu rogaviśeṣavijñānaṃ bhavati; tadyathā – āptopadeśaḥ pratyakṣam anumānaṃ ceti.* See also, e.g., Biardeau 1964: 446 f., Filliozat 1968: 440, Roşu 1978b: 88 and Filliozat 1990: 33.

[136]See *CS Vi* 4.5: [...] *trividhe tv asmin jñānasamudaye pūrvam āptopadeśāj jñānam, tataḥ pratyakṣānumānābhyāṃ parīkṣopapadyate. kiṃ hy anupadiṣṭaṃ pūrvaṃ yat tat pratyakṣānumānābhyāṃ parīkṣamāṇo vidyāt. tasmād dvividhā parīkṣā jñānavatām – pratyakṣam anumānaṃ ca; trividhā vā sahopadeśena.* On this, see also, e.g., Filliozat 1968: 441 and Hedge 1976: 18.

[137]See *CS Vi* 4.6 for instruction, 4.7 for sense perception and inference, and 4.8, where further medically relevant matters and conditions which are primarily known by means of inference are added. For a translation of the sequence *CS Vi* 4.3–8 see also Chattopadhyaya 1977: 89–92.

[138]See *CS Vi* 4.7: [...] *pratyakṣato 'numānād upadeśataś ca parīkṣaṇam uktam.* This may be also the reason for the identical order of the three means of knowledge enumerated in *Śā* 6.28 where the implicit context is provided by the examination of patients for signs of longevity or their opposite. However, depending on the interpretation of the expression

Vi 8.83 means of examination (*parīkṣā*)	*Vi* 4.3 means of in-depth knowledge of specific diseases (*rogaviśeṣajñāna*)	*Vi* 4.5, 7 means of examination (*parīkṣā, parīkṣaṇa*)
sense perception (*pratyakṣa*)	instruction by trustworthy persons (*āptopadeśa*)	sense perception (*pratyakṣa*)
inference (*anumāna*)	sense perception (*pratyakṣa*)	inference (*anumāna*)
+ instruction (*upadeśa*)	inference (*anumāna*)	+ instruction (*upadeśa*)

Table 3.19: The "2+1 Model" of Means of Knowledge in the *Carakasaṃhitā*

of knowledge can thus be presented as in Table 3.19.

The "2 + 1 model" may actually be a modernization and streamlining of the model of four sources of knowledge presented in *CS Sū* 11 (see Table 3.16 above) because some unspecified notion of *yukti* appears to be integrated as an essential factor of inference in the characterization of inference in *CS Vi* 4,[139] a characterization which found its way almost *verbatim* into the *vāda* section of *CS Vi* 8 as the char-

"all bodies of expert knowledge" (*sarvatantra*), this order may just follow the usual one established elsewhere. See *CS Śā* 6.28: *pratyakṣānumānopadeśāś cāpramāṇāni syur ye pramāṇabhūtāḥ sarvatantreṣu yair āyuṣyāṇy anāyuṣyāṇi copalabhyante.*

[139]See *CS Vi* 4.4: [...] *anumānaṃ khalu tarko yuktyapekṣaḥ.* On this, see also Hedge 1976: 18, Roşu 1978b: 84 and Filliozat 1990: 38.

acterization of inference as *pada* no. 20.[140] The order of the (remaining) three items in *Vi* 4.3 may still reflect the order as found in the metaphysical context of the *paralokaiṣaṇā* section of *CS Sū* 11, even though for identical contextual reasons, i.e., to acknowledge the progressive application in the practical, clinical context, it was changed in *Vi* 4.5 and 7 as well as in the short passage *Vi* 8.83.[141]

We can thus conclude that the *Carakasaṃhitā* offers us three epistemological models[142] indicative of the observational–rational attitude of early classical Indian medicine;[143] even though one of them, the model found in the *vāda* section of *CS Vi* 8, may have been taken over from another, possibly non-medical source, its explanations and exemplifications point to their origin in the medical setting, and this judgement therefore also applies to it. None of these three models precisely matches the model known from the *Nyāyasūtra*,[144] i.e., exactly mirrors the number and order of knowledge sources and the terminology employed in their proper designation, characterization and division. In addition to Table 3.20 below (see p. 121), figures visualiz-

---

[140]See *CS Vi* 8.42 (crit. ed.) (on this new numbering of the established text segments of *CS Vi* 8, see above, p. 82): *anumānaṃ nāma tarko yuktyapekṣaḥ* [...].

[141]On the possible motives for this order in *CS Śā* 6.28, see n. 138 above.

[142]On the various schemes of means of knowledge in the *Carakasaṃhitā*, though interpreted in a different, synthetic manner, see also Hedge 1976. For a synthetic and ahistorical approach to the topic of means of knowledge in Ayurveda, with frequent references to the relevant passages in the *Carakasaṃhitā* (as well as other classical works) and consideration of the practical relevance for practitioners of Ayurveda, see, e.g., the exposition in Narasimhacharyulu's text book written to comply with the C.C.I.M. syllabus (Narasimhacharyulu 2004: 189–344).

[143]See Roşu 1978b: 77 f. with reference to the distinction of three "schools" of Hippocratic medicine: philosophical, practical and observational–rational with scientific intentions.

[144]See n. 111 above.

ing the criss-cross of terminological correspondences, similar to the one presented above for the concepts of "instruction by trustworthy persons" and "verbal testimony" (see Figure 3.3), would make this aspect and the complex relationship between all these models and their variants more than clear.

The model that comes closest to the model of the *Nyāyasūtra* from one point of view may be the one found in the *vāda* section of *CS Vi* 8, in the list of forty-four *pada*s together with the subsequent text segments devoted to the individual terms and items. This model includes comparison or analogy (*aupamya*), which – although regularly employed in medical reasoning – does not have a place in the other models.[145] The contextually problematic enumeration of four sources of knowledge as causes of cognition (*upalabdhihetu*) under the item *hetu* ("demonstration / statement of proof") in *Vi* 8.33,[146] which is also included in Table 3.20 below, is confirmed by the new critical edition of *CS Vi* 8 and comes even closer in this respect: sense perception is followed by inference, oral tradition (*aitihya*) and comparison/analogy (*aupamya*).[147] From other points of view, i.e., the terminology and order of the last two items, the enumeration in *CS Vi* 8.33 also differs from the model of the *Nyāyasūtra*; it is closer to the model of *CS Vi* 8.27 with regard to the term used for comparison/analogy, namely, *aupamya*, instead of *upamāna* in the *Nyāyasūtra*, and on account of the employment of the identical term *aitihya*, which, how-

[145]On this point see also Filliozat (1968: 440) who assumes that analogy was denied the status of an independent means of proof by the physicians.

[146]See also n. 54 above, and further n. 118.

[147]See *CS Vi* 8.33 (crit. ed.): *hetuḥ: hetur nāmopalabdhikāraṇam. tat pratyakṣam anumānam aitihyam aupamyam iti. ebhir hetubhir yad upalabhyate tat tattvam.* On *Vi* 8.33 see further Kang 2007: 55–63.

ever, at the same time points to a discrepancy between these two models because *aitihya* according to *CS Vi* 8.33 probably encompasses what is meant by the two separate items *śabda* and *aitihya* according to *CS Vi* 8.27, a point which moves the model of *CS Vi* 8.33 again closer to the *Nyāyasūtra* model, as does the order of the first two items in both these models and the overall number of the means of knowledge in them. All models addressed and treated above may be summarized as in Table 3.20.

The epistemological models found in the *Carakasaṃhitā* may be augmented by means of further materials from the classical medical literature. It may be pointed out that in the edited text of the *Suśrutasaṃhitā* (*SS*) four sources of knowledge are mentioned in still another, unusual order: sense perception, tradition (*āgama*), inference and comparison/analogy (*upamāna*).[148] The editor records here a variant reading to this order according to which tradition occupies the primary position,[149] a feature also to be noted in the otherwise diverging model of the *paralokaiṣaṇā* section of *CS Sū* 11 and the unmodified, initial sequence of the model of *CS Vi* 4 as found in text segment 4.3, although the model of *SS Sū* even according to this variant reading differs in other ways from both these models of the *Carakasaṃhitā*. Ḍalhaṇa comments on the first sequence as follows, unambiguously revealing an empiricist ideology: Tradition is more excellent because it is the result of perception; thus, the author, i.e., Dhanvantari, has specified it before inference.[150] The *Aṣṭāṅgasaṅgraha*, however, records a statement of Suśruta in

[148]See *SS Sū* 1.16: *tasya* (scil. *āyurvedasya*) *aṅgavaram ādyaṃ pratyakṣāgamānumānopamānair aviruddham ucyamānam upadhāraya*.

[149]See n. 2: *āgamapratyakṣānumānopamānaiḥ* instead of *pratyakṣāgamānumānopamānaiḥ*.

[150]See *Nibandhasaṅgraha* (*NiS*) 4b, 9f.: *āgamasya pratyakṣaphalatvād varīyastvam. tenānumānāt pūrvaṃ nirdiṣṭavān*. The statement seems to imply

CS Sū 11.17 means of examination/ knowledge (*parīkṣā*, *pramāṇa*)	*CS Vi* 4.3 means of in-depth knowledge of specific diseases (*rogaviśeṣa-jñāna*)	*CS Vi* 4.5, 7 means of examination (*parīkṣā*, *parīkṣaṇa*)	*CS Vi* 8.83 means of examination (*parīkṣā*)	*CS Śā* 6.28 means of knowledge (*pramāṇa*)	*CS Vi* 8.27 items (*padas*) no. 17–21 (see p. 82 above)	*CS Vi* 8.33 division of item (*pada*) no. 11 (*hetu*)	*NS* 1.1.3 means of knowledge (*pramāṇa*)
instruction by trustworthy persons (*āptopadeśa*; *āptāgama*)	instruction by trustworthy persons (*āptopadeśa*)	sense perception (*pratyakṣa*)	sense perception (*pratyakṣa*)	sense perception (*pratyakṣa*)	verbal testimony (*śabda*)	sense perception (*pratyakṣa*)	sense perception (*pratyakṣa*)
sense perception (*pratyakṣa*)	sense perception (*pratyakṣa*)	inference (*anumāna*)	inference (*anumāna*)	inference (*anumāna*)	sense perception (*pratyakṣa*)	inference (*anumāna*)	inference (*anumāna*)
inference (*anumāna*)	inference (*anumāna*)	+ instruction (*upadeśa*)	+ instruction (*upadeśa*)	instruction (*upadeśa*)	comparison/ analogy (*aupamya*)	oral tradition (*aitihya*)	comparison/ analogy (*upamāna*)
yukti					oral tradition (*aitihya*)	comparison/ analogy (*aupamya*)	verbal testimony (*śabda*)
					inference (*anumāna*)		

Table 3.20: Epistemological Models in the *Carakasaṃhitā* and *Nyāyasūtra*

which he mentions only three means of knowledge, namely, tradition (*āgama*), sense perception and inference, in this order, as in the model of *CS Vi* 4.3.[151]

As regards the determination of the individual knowledge sources according to the various models under the aspect of their precise nature, merely a first start in this direction has been made above with the analytic, mainly structural examination of "instruction by trustworthy persons" and "verbal testimony" (see 3.2.4).

3.2.7 From the above exposition, elaboration and discussion of Vidyabhusana's original hypothesis on the early development of Indian logic (see Figures 3.1 and 3.2 above) with the help of some examples taken from the area of dialectics and epistemology, and with only very few selected references to other (early) classical sources for our knowledge of these areas, it should have become obvious that in spite of a number of resemblances with varying degree of closeness and of various kinds (to which further ones could be added), the evidence offered by the *Carakasaṃhitā* is far too varied and complex in itself to allow a definite and precise determination of the interesting and certainly intriguing relationship in the area of dialectics and epistemology between this earliest classical medical Saṃhitā and the later *Nyāyasūtra*, or rather the traditional background of the latter work, namely, the hypothetical Nyāyaśāstra and a certain part of the still earlier Ānvīkṣikī assigned to Medhā-

that *anumāna*, as a less excellent source of knowledge, is the result not only of perception, but also of some other factor(s).

[151]See *AS Sū* 20, p. 193a, 18–20 (= *Sū* 20.18 according to the Āṭhavale 1980 edition): *suśrutaḥ punaḥ paṭhati: ... tad evam etāni vāyvādirūpakarmāṇy avahitaḥ samyag upalakṣayed āgamapratyakṣānumānaiḥ*. I owe this reference to Dr Ernst Prets, Vienna.

tithi Gautama (which both would have to be reconstructed on the way), as was suggested by Vidyabhusana.

In the forthcoming continuation and conclusion of this paper (Part II), the diametrically opposed hypothesis by Surendranath Dasgupta will be presented, discussed and evaluated, followed by further references to the most important scholarship outside India and in more recent times on the issue, and some methodological considerations concerning future research into it.

Appendix

Some Notes on the Earliest Edition of the *Carakasaṃhitā*

Roth (1872: 441 f.), mentions Gangadhar Kaviraj's edition published in 1868 as the first attempt to edit the text. It was published in fascicles by the Samvadajnanaratnakara Press, Kolkata, in Bengali and Nagari letters; the year of the actual completion of this first edition remains to be documented. In 1878, it was republished (and possibly completed) by Dharanidhar Ray Kaviraj in Berhampore, Saidabad (Pramadabhanjana Press).[152] In the extensive bibliography of editions of the *Carakasaṃhitā* listed in Meulenbeld 1999: IB, pp. 3–6, both editions are mentioned under "c" (p. 3).

The earliest edition according to this bibliography, i.e., the edition by Narendranath Sengupta and Balaichandra Sengupta (Calcutta 1849–1855), which was not seen by Meulenbeld (p. 3, labelled "*a"), is actually an edition which appeared in 1927–1933 and is identical with Meulenbeld's edition "w" (p. 4 f.).[153] Evidently the *śaka* years were mistaken for years of the Common Era.

---

[152]See also CS[SGAS]: 14 f., item no. 3 where, however, the date of publication of the second volume [*saṃ* 1971, i.e., 1914] must be wrong.

[153]See also CS[SGAS]: 14 f., item no. 2.

The second-oldest edition mentioned by Meulenbeld (p. 3) is an edition by a certain Shankar Shastri, published by the Nirnaya Sagar Press, Mumbai, in 1867 (labelled "*b"); in Preisendanz 2007: 635, n. 39, I still considered this edition to be the *editio princeps*. However, as was noticed by Dr Philipp A. Maas, one of my colleagues in the projects mentioned in the acknowledgements note on p. 63 above, the date 1867 appearing on the title page of the book is *not* the date of publication of this edition, but refers to the year when the copyright law applying to it was passed. The book is obviously a re-edition – without the Marathi translation and notes – of Shankar Daji Shastri Pade's edition by his son Shankar Shastri; the original was published in fourteen fascicles in Mumbai from 1897 to 1898 by the bookseller Yajneshvar Gopal Dikshit (Meulenbeld's "i²," p. 3). For some unknown reason, Meulenbeld, who did not see *b, refers under this item to "ed. Poona 1926," a reprint of this 1897–1898 edition with translation, published in 1926 by the same bookseller, now located in Pune, and printed in Pune at the Hanuman Press; it was edited by Krishna Shastri Kavade.[154]

The original of the copy of *b available to the abovementioned projects is owned by the library of the Institute for South Asian and Central Asian Studies, University of Leipzig, Germany, and was part of the personal library of the late Friedrich Weller (call number W/Fae 2); it does not contain a date of publication.[155] However, in the library's card catalogue the date of publication is given as 1903. Interestingly, the old card catalogue of the library of the Karl Sudhoff Institute for the History of Medicine, University of

[154]See also CS[SGAS]: 16 f., item no. 13.

[155]See also the undated Nirnaya Sagar Press edition by Shankara Shastrin referred to in Filliozat 1993: 104, n. 13.

Leipzig, also refers to an edition of the *Carakasaṃhitā* published from Bombay in 1903; the editor is said to be a certain Candaravastrin, a strange name indeed. In early 2009, the book (call number II 8253) could not be located on the shelves; however, it may eventually be found to be identical with the other Leipzig copy (i.e., W/Fae 2), and "Candaravastrin" may go back to a (faulty or illegible) transliteration of the reference to the editor "Śaṅkara Śāstrin" on the Devanāgarī-script title page of the book.

Abbreviations and Sigla

ĀD	*Āyurvedadīpikā*. See Ācārya 1941.
AŚ	*Arthaśāstra*. See Kangle 1960.
AS	*Aṣṭāṅgasaṅgraha*. See Chhanganee 1991.
ASBh	*Abhidharmasamuccayabhāṣya*. See Tatia 1976.
BṛU	*Bṛhadāraṇyaka-Upaniṣad*. See Olivelle 1998.
CS	*Carakasaṃhitā*. See Ācārya 1941.
CS (crit. ed.)	*Carakasaṃhitā (crit. ed.)*. See Preisendanz *et al.* in preparation.
CS[SGAS]	*Carakasaṃhitā* (Shri Gulabkunverba ed., v. 1). See Mehta 1949.
DCSSUV	*Descriptive Catalogue...Varanasi*. See Sarasvati Bhavana Library 1996.
GPBh	*Gauḍapādabhāṣya*. See Esnoul 1964.
JM	*Jayamaṅgalā*. See Sharma and Vangiya 1970.
NĀA	*Nyāyāgamānusāriṇī*. See Jambuvijayaji 1966.
NBh	*Nyāyabhāṣya*. See Thakur 1997a.
NiS	*Nibandhasaṅgraha*. See Ācārya 1938.
NM II	*Nyāyamañjarī*. See Varadacarya 1983.
NS	*Nyāyasūtra*. See Ruben 1928.
NV	*Nyāyavārttika*. See Thakur 1997b.
P	*Pāṇini*. See Böhtlingk 1887.
PSV	*Pramāṇasamuccayavṛtti*. See Suzuki 1957.
PT	*Pañcatantra*. See Kale 1912.
PV	*Pramāṇavārttika*. See Sankrityayana 1938–1940.
Śā	*Śārīrasthāna*
SāS	*Sārasaṅgraha*. See Dvivedi 1903.
SK	*Sāṅkhyakārikā*. See Wezler and Motegi 1998, Esnoul 1964.
SS	*Suśrutasaṃhitā*. See Ācārya 1938.

ŚU	*Śvetāśvatara-Upaniṣad*. See Olivelle 1998.
Sū	*Sūtrasthāna*
TS	*Tattvasaṅgraha* of Śāntarakṣita. See Shastri 1968.
Vi	*Vimānasthāna*
**VP*	*Vaidalyaprakaraṇa*. See Tola and Dragonetti 1995.
YD	*Yuktidīpikā*. See Wezler and Motegi 1998.
YP	*Yatidharmaprakāśa*. See Olivelle 1976–1977.

References

Ācārya, Yādavaśarman Trivikrama (ed.) 1938. *Suśrutasaṃhitā, Suśrutena viracitā, VaidyavaraśrīḌalhaṇācāryaviracitayā Nibandhasaṃgrahākhyavyākhyayā samullasitā, Ācāryopāhvena Trivikramātmajena Yādavaśarmaṇṇā saṃśodhitā*. Mumbayyāṃ: Nirṇayasāgara Mudrāyantrālaye, 3rd edn.

— 1941. *Maharṣiṇā Punarvasunopadiṣṭā, tacchiṣyeṇāgniveśena praṇītā, CarakaDṛḍhabalābhyāṃ pratisaṃskṛtā Carakasaṃhitā, śrīCakrapāṇidattaviracitayā āyurvedadīpikāvyākhyayā saṃvalitā*. Mumbayyāṃ: Nirṇayasāgara Mudrāyantrālaye, 3rd edn.

Āṭhavale, Anaṃta Dāmodara (ed.) 1980. *Aṣṭāṅgasaṅgrahaḥ. ŚrīmadVṛddhavāgbhaṭaviracitaḥ Induvyākhyāsahitaḥ*. Puṇe: Maheśa Anaṃta Āṭhavale, Śrīmad Ātreya Prakāśanam.

Aufrecht, Theodor 1869. *A Catalogue of Sanskrit Manuscripts in the Library of Trinity College, Cambridge*. Cambridge and London: Deighton, Bell, & co.

Balcerowicz, Piotr 2001. *Jaina Epistemology in Historical and Comparative Perspective. Critical Edition and English Translation of Logical–Epistemological Treatises: Nyāyâvatāra, Nyāyâvatāra-vivṛti and Nyāyâvatāra-ṭippaṇa with Introduction and Notes*, vol. 53 of *Alt- und Neu-Indische Studien*. Stuttgart: Franz Steiner Verlag.

Biardeau, Madeleine 1964. *Théorie de la connaissance et philosophie de la parole dans le brahmanisme classique*, vol. 23 of *Le monde d'outre-mer passé et présent, première série, études*. Paris and La Haye: Mouton.

Böhtlingk, Otto 1883–1886. *Sanskrit-Wörterbuch in kürzerer Fassung*. St. Petersburg: Buchdruckerei der Kaiserlichen Akademie der Wissenschaften. 7v.

— 1887. *Pāṇini's Grammatik*. Leipzig: Haessel, 2nd edn.

Chakravarti, Chintaharan 1929–1930. "Bengal's Contribution to Sanskrit Literature (A Chronological Framework)." *Annals of the Bhandarkar Oriental Research Institute*, **11**, 234–58.

Chattopadhyay, Rita 1995. *Gaṅgādhara Kavirāja: A 19th Century Polymath in Oblivion*. Calcutta: Sanskrit Pustak Bhandar.

Chattopadhyaya, Debiprasad 1977. *Science and Society in Ancient India*. Calcutta: Research India Publications.

Chhanganee, Govardhansharma (ed.) 1991. *Aṣṭāṅgasaṅgraha (Sūtrasthānam) by Shrimad-Bagbhatacharya (Based on Old Bagbhat) with Excellent 'Asthaprakashika' Commentaries*, vol. 157 of *Kashi Sanskrit Series*. Varanasi, 7th edn.

Comba, Antonella 1987. "Carakasaṃhitā, Śārīrasthāna I and Vaiśeṣika Philosophy." In G. Jan Meulenbeld and Dominik Wujastyk (eds.), *Studies on Indian Medical History. Papers Presented at the International Workshop on the Study of Indian Medicine Held at the Wellcome Institute for the History of Medicine 2–4 September 1985*, vol. 2 of *Groningen Oriental Studies*, pp. 39–55. Groningen: Egbert Forsten.

— 1990. "Universal (*sāmānya*) and Particular (*viśeṣa*) in Vaiśeṣika and Āyurveda." *Journal of the European Āyurvedic Society*, **1**, 7–32.

Das, Rahul Peter 1993. "Heilskonzepte in der altindischen ('hinduistischen') Medizin." In Klaus Giel and Renate

Breuninger (eds.), *Religionen und medizinische Ethik*, vol. 7 of *Bausteine zur Philosophie*, pp. 11–40. Ulm: Universität Ulm Humboldt-Studienzentrum.

Dasgupta, Surendranath 1922. *A History of Indian Philosophy. Vol. II*. Cambridge: Cambridge University Press.

Dvivedi, Vindyeshvari Prasad (ed.) 1903. *Tārkikarakṣā śrīmadācāryavaradarājaviracitā tatkṛtasārasaṅgrahābhidhavyākhyāsahitā*. Varanasi: Meḍikalhālnāmakayantrālaye, 2nd edn.

Eggeling, Julius 1896. *Catalogue of the Sanskrit Manuscripts in the Library of the India Office. Vol. I, Part 5*. London: Printed by order of the Secretary of State for India in Council.

Esnoul, Anne-Marie 1964. *Les strophes de Sāṃkhya (Sāṃkhya-Kārikā) avec le commentaire de Gauḍapāda. Texte Sanskrit et traduction annotée*. Collection Émile Senart. Paris: Société d'édition «Les Belles Lettres».

Filliozat, Jean 1968. "Langues et littératures de L'Inde. I. L'esprit de la science indienne (suite): Le raisonnement et la discussion en médecine." *Annuaire du Collège de France*, **68**, 439–43.

Filliozat, Pierre-Sylvain 1990. "*Yukti*, le quatrième *pramāṇa* des médecins (Carakasaṃhitā, Sūtrasthāna XI, 25)." *Journal of the European Āyurvedic Society*, **1**, 33–46.

— 1993. "Caraka's Proof of Rebirth." *Journal of the European Āyurvedic Society*, **3**, 94–111.

Frauwallner, Erich 1958. "Die Erkenntnislehre des klassischen Sāṃkhya-Systems." *Wiener Zeitschrift für die Kunde Süd- und Ostasiens*, **2**, 84–139.

— 1984. "Erkenntnistheorie und Logik der klassischen Zeit." In Ernst Steinkellner (ed.), *Nachgelassene Werke I. Aufsätze, Beiträge, Skizzen*, vol. 438 of *Österreichische Akademie der Wissenschaften, philosophisch-historische Klasse, Sitzungsberichte*, pp. 66–87. Wien: Österreichische

Akademie der Wissenschaften.

Garbe, Richard 1899. *Verzeichnis der indischen Handschriften der königlichen Universitäts-Bibliothek (Zuwachs der Jahre 1865–1899). Verzeichnis der Doktoren, welche die philosophische Fakultät der königlich Württembergischen Eberhard-Karls-Universität in Tübingen im Dekanatsjahre 1898–1899 ernannt hat*. (Supplement). Tübingen: Laupp.

Gupta, Brahmananda 1976. "Indigenous Medicine in Nineteeth- and Twentieth-century Bengal." In Charles Leslie (ed.), *Asian Medical Systems. A Comparative Study*, pp. 368–78. Berkeley: University of California Press. Reprinted Delhi: Motilal Banarsidass, 1998.

Halbfass, Wilhelm 1992. *On Being and What There Is. Classical Vaiśeṣika and the History of Indian Ontology*. Albany: State University of New York Press.

Hedge, R. D. 1976. "Caraka's Concept of Pramāṇa." *Mysore Orientalist*, **9**, 17–21.

Jambuvijayaji, Muni (ed.) 1966. *Dvādaśāraṃ Nayacakraṃ of Ācārya Śrī Mallavādi Kṣamāśramaṇa With the Commentary Nyāyāgamānusāriṇī of Śrī Siṃhasūri Gaṇi Vādi Kṣamāśramaṇa. Part I (1–4 Aras)*, vol. 92 of *Śrī Ātmānand Jain Granthamālā*. Bhavnagar: Jaina Atmananda Sabha.

Kale, M. R. (ed.) 1912. *Pañcatantra of Viṣṇuśarman*. Bombay (Reprint Delhi 1986).

Kang, Sung Yong 2003. *Die Debatte im alten Indien. Untersuchungen zum Sambhāṣāvidhi und verwandten Themen in der Carakasaṃhitā Vimānasthāna 8.15–28*, vol. 6 of *Philosophica Indica – Einsichten · Ansichten*. Reinbek: Dr. Inge Wezler Verlag für Orientalistische Fachpublikationen.

— 2007. *Pañcāvayava: Die fünfgliedrige Argumentationsform in den frühen Debattentraditionen Indiens mit besonderer Berücksichtigung der Carakasaṃhitā Vi. 8.30–36*. Göttingen: Cuvillier.

— 2009. "What does *-sama* Mean? On the Uniform Ending of the Names of the *jāti*-s in the *Nyāyasūtra*." *Journal of Indian Philosophy*, **37,1**, 75–96.

Kangle, R. P. (ed.) 1960. *Arthaśāstra. The Kauṭilīya Arthaśāstra. Part I. A Critical Edition with a Glossary*, vol. 1 of *University of Bombay Studies – Sanskrit, Prakrit and Pali*. Bombay: University of Bombay.

Larson, Gerald James 1987. "Āyurveda and the Hindu Philosophical Systems." *Philosophy East and West*, **37,3**, 245–59.

Maas, Philipp A. 2010a. "Computer Aided Stemmatics – The Case of Fifty-Two Text Versions of Carakasaṃhitā Vimānasthāna 8.67–157." *Wiener Zeitschrift für die Kunde Südasiens*, **52–53**, 63–119.

— 2010b. "On What Became of the Carakasaṃhitā After Dṛḍhabala's Revision." *eJournal of Indian Medicine*, **3**, 1–22.

Mehta, P. M. (ed.) 1949. *The Caraka Saṃhitā Expounded by the Worshipful Ātreya Punarvasu, Compiled by the Great Sage Agniveśa and Redacted by Caraka & Dṛḍhabala. Edited and Published in 6 Volumes with Translations in Hindi, Gujarati and English by Shree Gulabkunverba Ayurvedic Society*. Jamnagar: The Society. 6v.

Meindersma, Tabe E. 1990. "*Paralokasiddhi* in *Carakasaṃhitā*." *Indologica Taurinensia*, **15–16**, 265–73.

— 1992. "Caraka and the Materialists." *Wiener Zeitschrift für die Kunde Südasiens (Supplement)*, **36**, 299–306.

Meisig, Konrad (ed.) 1994. *Rudolf von Roth. Kleine Schriften*, vol. 36 of *Glasenapp-Stiftung*. Stuttgart.

Meulenbeld, G. Jan 1999. *A History of Indian Medical Literature. Vol. IA: Text, Vol. IB: Annotation*, vol. XV of *Groningen Oriental Studies*. Groningen: Egbert Forsten.

Narain, Harsh 1976. *Evolution of the Nyāya–Vaiśeṣika Categoriology*. Varanasi: Bharati Prakashan.

Narasimhacharyulu, K. V. L. 2004. *Padārtha Vijñāna*, vol. 101 of *Krishnadas Ayurveda Series*. Varanasi: Chaukhambha Sanskrit Sansthan.

Oberhammer, Gerhard 1963. "Ein Beitrag zu den Vāda-Traditionen." *Wiener Zeitschrift für die Kunde Süd- und Ostasiens*, **7**, 63–103.

— 1991. *Terminologie der frühen philosophischen Scholastik in Indien. Ein Begriffswörterbuch zur altindischen Dialektik, Erkenntnislehre und Methodologie. Band 1: A–I*, vol. 223 of *Österreichische Akademie der Wissenschaften, philosophisch-historische Klasse, Denkschriften*. Wien: Österreichische Akademie der Wissenschaften.

Oberhammer, Gerhard, Ernst Prets, and Joachim Prandstetter 2006. *Terminologie der frühen philosophischen Scholastik in Indien. Ein Begriffswörterbuch zur altindischen Dialektik, Erkenntnislehre und Methodologie. Band 3: Pra–H*, vol. 343 of *Österreichische Akademie der Wissenschaften, philosophisch-historische Klasse, Denkschriften*. Wien: Österreichische Akademie der Wissenschaften.

Oberlies, Thomas 1995. "Die Śvetāśvatara-Upaniṣad: Einleitung, Edition und Übersetzung von Adhyāya I." *Wiener Zeitschrift für die Kunde Südasiens*, **39**, 61–201.

Oetke, Claus 1994. *Vier Studien zum altindischen Syllogismus*, vol. 2 of *Philosophica Indica – Einsichten · Ansichten*. Reinbek: Dr. Inge Wezler Verlag für Orientalistische Fachpublikationen.

Olivelle, Patrick 1976–1977. *Vāsudevāśrama Yatidharmaprakāśa: a Treatise on World Renunciation*, vol. 3–4 of *Publications of the De Nobili Research Library*. Vienna: Sammlung De Nobili.

— 1998. *The Early Upaniṣads. Annotated Text and Translation.* New York and Oxford: Oxford University Press.

Pecchia, Cristina 2010. "Transmission-specific (In)utility, or Dealing with Contamination: Samples from the Textual Tradition of the Carakasaṃhitā." *Wiener Zeitschrift für die Kunde Südasiens*, **52–53**, 121–59.

Pind, Ole Holten 2001. "Why the Vaidalyaprakaraṇa Cannot Be an Authentic Work of Nāgārjuna." *Wiener Zeitschrift für die Kunde Südasiens / Vienna Journal of South Asian Studies*, **45**, 149–72.

Preisendanz, Karin 1994. *Studien zu Nyāyasūtra III.1 mit dem Nyāyatattvāloka Vācaspati Miśras II*, vol. 46 of *Alt- und Neu-Indische Studien*. Stuttgart: Franz Steiner Verlag.

— 2000 [2001]. "Debate and Independent Reasoning vs. Tradition: On the Precarious Position of Early Nyāya." In Ryutaro Tsuchida and Albrecht Wezler (eds.), *Harānandalaharī. Volume in Honour of Professor Minoru Hara on his Seventieth Birthday*, pp. 221–51. Reinbek: Dr. Inge Wezler Verlag für Orientalistische Fachpublikationen.

— 2007. "The Initiation of the Medical Student in Early Classical Āyurveda: Caraka's Treatment in Context." In B. Kellner *et al.* (eds.), *Pramāṇakīrtiḥ. Papers Dedicated to Ernst Steinkellner on the Occasion of his 70th Birthday*, vol. 70 of *Wiener Studien zur Tibetologie und Buddhismuskunde*, pp. 629–68. Wien: Arbeitskreis für Tibetische und Buddhistische Studien.

— 2010. "Reasoning as a Science, its Role in Early Dharma Literature, and the Emergence of the Term *nyāya*." In Brendan S. Gillon (ed.), *Logic in Earliest Classical India*, vol. 10.2 of *Papers of the 12th World Sanskrit Conference* (ed. by Petteri Koskikallio and Asko Parpola), pp. 27–66. Delhi: Motilal Banarsidass.

Preisendanz, Karin, Cristina Pecchia, and Philipp A. Maas

(eds.) in preparation. Text of the Carakasaṃhitā Vimānasthāna as critically edited by the "Philosophy and Medicine in Early Classical India" projects at the University of Vienna.

Prets, Ernst 1994. "The Structure of *sādhana* in the Abhidharmasamuccaya." *Wiener Zeitschrift für die Kunde Südasiens*, **38**, 337–50.

— 2004. "Example and Examplification in Early Nyāya and Vaiśeṣika." In Shoryu Katsura and Ernst Steinkellner (eds.), *The Role of the Example (Dṛṣṭānta) in Classical Indian Logic*, vol. 58 of *Wiener Studien zur Tibetologie und Buddhismuskunde*, pp. 197–224. Wien: Arbeitskreis für Tibetische und Buddhistische Studien.

— 2010. "On the Proof Passage of the *Carakasaṃhitā*: Editions, Manuscripts and Commentaries." In Brendan S. Gillon (ed.), *Logic in Earliest Classical India*, vol. 10.2 of *Papers of the 12th World Sanskrit Conference* (ed. by Petteri Koskikallio and Asko Parpola), pp. 67–85. Delhi: Motilal Banarsidass.

Randle, H. N. 1926. "Review of Vidyabhusana 1921." *Mind*, **35**, 84–87 ("Critical Notices").

Roşu, Arion 1978a. "Études āyurvédiques: le *trivarga* dans l'āyurveda." *Indologica Taurinensia*, **6**, 255–60.

— 1978b. *Les conceptions psychologiques dans les textes médicaux indiens*, vol. 43 of *Publications de l'Institut de Civilisation Indienne Série in-8*. Paris: Institut de Civilisation Indienne.

Roth, Rudolf 1872. "Indische Medicin. Caraka." *Zeitschrift der Deutschen Morgenländischen Gesellschaft*, **26**, 441–52. Reprinted in Meisig 1994: 467–78.

Ruben, Walter 1928. *Die Nyāyasūtra's. Text, Übersetzung, Erläuterung und Glossar*, vol. 18.2 of *Abhandlungen für die Kunde des Morgenlandes*. Leipzig: Deutsche Morgenländische Gesellschaft.

Sankrityayana, Rahula (ed.) 1938–1940. *Dharmakīrti's Pramāṇavārttika with a Commentary by Manorathanandin.* Patna: Bihar and Orissa Research Society. Published as an appendix to vols. 24–26 of the *Journal of the Bihar and Orissa Research Society.*

Sarasvati Bhavana Library 1996. *A Descriptive Catalogue of the Sanskrit Manuscripts Acquired for and Deposited in the Sampurnanand Sanskrit University Library (Sarasvati Bhavana), Varanasi During the Years 1951–1981*, vol. 12.2 of *A Descriptive Catalogue of the Sanskrit Manuscripts Acquired for and Deposited in the Sanskrit University Library (Sarasvati Bhavana), Varanasi During the Years 1791–1950.* Varanasi: Dr. Harish Chandra Mani Tripathi.

Scharfe, Hartmut 1989. *The State in Indian Tradition*, vol. II.3.2 of *Handbuch der Orientalistik.* Leiden etc.: Brill.

Scharfstein, Ben-Ami 1997. "The Three Philosophical Traditions." In Eli Franco and Karin Preisendanz (eds.), *Beyond Orientalism. The Work of Wilhelm Halbfass and its Impact on Indian and Cross-Cultural Studies*, vol. 59 of *Poznań Studies in the Philosophy of the Sciences and the Humanities*, pp. 235–95. Amsterdam and Atlanta: Rodopi.

— 1998. *A Comparative History of World Philosophy: From the Upanishads to Kant.* New York: State University of New York Press.

Scherrer-Schaub, Cristina 1981. "Le terme *yukti*: première étude." *Asiatische Studien / Études Asiatiques*, **35**, 185–99.

Sharma, Priya Vrat 1994. *Caraka-Saṃhitā. Agniveśa's Treatise Refined and Annotated by Caraka and Redacted by Dṛḍhabala (Text with English Translation). Vol. 1*, vol. 36 of *Jaikrishnadas Ayurveda Series.* Varanasi and Delhi: Chaukhamba Orientalia, 3rd edn.

Sharma, Ram Karan and Bhagwan Dash 1994. *Agnivesa's*

Caraka Saṃhitā (Text with English Translation & Critical Exposition Based on Cakrapani Datta's Ayurvedadipika), vol. II, vol. 94 of *Chowkhamba Sanskrit Studies.* Varanasi: Chowkhamba Sanskrit Series Office.

Sharma, Vishnu Prasad and Satkarisharma Vangiya (eds.) 1970. *Sāṃkhyakārikā of Śrīmad Īśvarakṛṣṇa ... and the Jayamaṅgalā of Śrī Śaṅkara,* vol. 296 of *Chowkhamba Sanskrit Series.* Varanasi: Chowkhamba Sanskrit Series Office, 2nd edn.

Shastri, Swami Dwarikadas (ed.) 1968. *Tattvasaṅgraha of Ācārya Shāntarakṣita with the Commentary 'Pañjikā' of Shri Kamalashīla,* vol. 1 of *Bauddha Bharati Series.* Varanasi: Bauddha Bharati.

Solomon, Esther A. 1974. *The Commentaries of the Sāṃkhya Kārikā – A Study.* Ahmedabad: Gujarat University.

— 1976. *Indian Dialectics. Methods of Philosophical Discussion. Vol. I,* vol. 70 of *Research Series.* Ahmedabad: Sheth Bholabhai Jeshingbhai Institute of Learning and Research, Gujarat Vidya Sabha.

Steinkellner, Ernst 1984. "Anmerkungen zu einer buddhistischen Texttradition: Paralokasiddhi." *Anzeiger der Österreichischen Akademie der Wissenschaften, philosophisch-historische Klasse,* **121(4)**, 79–94.

von Stietencron, Heinrich 2003. "Attraktion und Ausstrahlung: Das Wirken Rudolf von Roths." In Heidrun Brückner *et al.* (eds.), *Indienforschung im Zeitenwandel. Analysen und Dokumente zur Indologie und Religionswissenschaft in Tübingen,* pp. 77–90. Tübingen: Attempto Verlag.

Suzuki, Daisetz Teitaro (ed.) 1957. *Pramāṇasamuccayavṛtti of Dignāga (Tshad ma kun las btus pa'i 'grel pa), Translation by Vasudhararakṣita and Seṅ rgyal,* vol. 130, no. 5701 of *The Tibetan Tripitaka, Peking Edition. Edited by Daisetz Teitaro Suzuki.* Tokyo, Kyoto: Tibetan Tripitaka Research

Institute.

Takakusu, J. 1904. "La Sāṃkhyakārikā étudiée à la lumière de sa version chinoise." *Bulletin de l'École Française d'Extrême-Orient*, **4**, 1–65 and 978–1064.

Tatia, Nathmal (ed.) 1976. *Abhidharmasamuccayabhāṣyam*, vol. 17 of *Tibetan Sanskrit Works Series*. Pāṭaliputram: Kāśīprasāda Jāyasavāla-Anuśīlana-Saṃsthā.

Thakur, Anantalal (ed.) 1997a. *Nyāyabhāṣya of Vātsyāyana*, in *Gautamīyanyāyadarśana with Bhāṣya of Vātsyāyana*, vol. 1 of *Nyāyacaturgranthikā*. New Delhi: Indian Council of Philosophical Research.

— 1997b. *Nyāyavārttika of Uddyotakara* in *Nyāyabhāṣyavārttika of Bhāradvāja Uddyotakara*, vol. 2 of *Nyāyacaturgranthikā*. New Delhi: Indian Council of Philosophical Research.

Tillemans, Tom J. F. 1984. "Sur le *parārthānumāna* en logique bouddhique." *Asiatische Studien / Études Asiatiques*, **38**, 73–98.

Tola, Fernando and Carmen Dragonetti 1995. *Nāgārjuna's Refutation of Logic (Nyāya). Vaidalyaprakaraṇa – Źib mo rnam par ḥthag pa ṣes bya baḥi rab tu byed pa. Edition of the Tibetan Text, English Translation and Commentary, With Introduction and Notes*, vol. 24 of *Buddhist Tradition Series*. Delhi: Motilal Banarsidass.

Tucci, Giuseppe 1930. *The Nyāyamukha of Dignāga. The Oldest Buddhist Text on Logic After Chinese and Tibetan Materials*, vol. 15 of *Materialien zur Kunde des Buddhismus*. Heidelberg: Institut für Buddhismuskunde.

Ui, H. 1917. *The Vais'eshesika Philosophy According to the Dasapadartha-Sastra: Chinese Text with Introduction, Translation and Notes*, vol. 24 of *Oriental Translation Fund, New Series*. London: Royal Asiatic Society.

Varadacarya, K. S. (ed.) 1983. *Nyāyamañjarī of Jayantabhaṭṭa with Ṭippaṇī Nyāyasaurabha by the Editor, vol. II*, vol. 139 of *University of Mysore Oriental Research Institute Series*. Mysore: University of Mysore Oriental Research Institute.

Vidyabhusana, Satis Chandra 1921. *A History of Indian Logic: Ancient, Mediaeval and Modern Schools*. Calcutta: Calcutta University. Reprinted: Delhi, Motilal Banarsidass, 1977, and often thereafter.

— 1930. *The Nyâya Sutras of Gotama Translated by M. M. Satîśa Chandra Vidyâbhuṣana, Revised and Enlarged by Nandalal Sinha*. Allahabad: The Pâṇini Office.

Vidyabhusana, Satis Chandra (ed., tr.) 1909. *Nyāyāvatāra: the Earliest Jaina Work on Pure Logic by Siddhasena Divākara with Sanskrit Text and Commentary*. Calcutta: The Indian Research Society.

Wezler, Albrecht 1994. "Credo, quia Occidentale: A Note on Sanskrit Varṇa and its Misinterpretation in Literature on Mīmāṃsā and Vyākaraṇa." In R. C. Dwivedi (ed.), *Studies in Mīmāṃsā. Dr. Mandan Mishra Felicitation Volume*, pp. 221–41. Delhi: Motilal Banarsidass.

Wezler, Albrecht and Shujun Motegi (eds.) 1998. *Yuktidīpikā. The Most Significant Commentary on the Sāṃkhyakārikā*, vol. 44 of *Alt- und Neu-Indische Studien*. Stuttgart: Franz Steiner Verlag.

Yoshimizu, Chizuko 1996. "Saṃdhinirmocanasūtra X ni okeru shishu no *yukti* ni tsuite" (On the four kinds of *yukti* in the tenth chapter of the Sandhinirmocanasūtra)." *Journal of the Naritasan Institute for Buddhist Studies*, **19**, 123–68.

— 2010. "The Logic of the *Saṃdhinirmocanasūtra*: Establishing Right Reasoning Based on Similarity (*sārupya*) and Dissimilarity (*vairūpya*)." In Brendan S. Gillon (ed.), *Logic in Earliest Classical India*, vol. 10.2 of *Papers of the 12th*

World Sanskrit Conference (ed. by Petteri Koskikallio and Asko Parpola), pp. 139–66. Delhi: Motilal Banarsidass.

Zeller, Gabriele 2003. "Rudolf von Roth als Schüler, Lehrer und Gelehrter." In Heidrun Brückner *et al.* (eds.), *Indienforschung im Zeitenwandel. Analysen und Dokumente zur Indologie und Religionswissenschaft in Tübingen*, pp. 91–118. Tübingen: Attempto Verlag.

4

DOMINIK WUJASTYK

New Manuscript Evidence for the Textual and Cultural History of Early Classical Indian Medicine

The importance of the *Suśrutasaṃhitā*

The *Suśrutasaṃhitā*, "The Compendium of Suśruta," is a world classic of the history of science. It was composed in South Asia, in the Sanskrit language, and its earliest content may date from as early as 250 BCE.[1] It was reedited several times until about CE 500, when the text achieved the general form in which we have it today.[2]

The *Suśrutasaṃhitā* was one of the defining texts for Ayurveda, the systematic and formal tradition of healing that became South Asia's principle medical system until the advent of modernity in the late eighteenth century.

Support for part of this research came from the Wellcome Trust under Wellcome Trust Senior Research Fellowship grant no. 066401.

[1]Third-century BCE grammatical sources refer to followers of a "Suśrut," though it is not certain that this is connected with the *Suśruta-saṃhitā* (the evidence is discussed by Meulenbeld 1999–2002: IA, 333 and IB, 435, n. 42). Medical narratives in the Buddhist Canon, also broadly datable to this period, are consistent with an early medical and surgical tradition that has strong parallels with the later *Carakasaṃhitā* and the *Suśrutasaṃhitā* (Zysk 1991: ch. 6).

[2]Meulenbeld 1999–2002: IA, 333–57, Wujastyk 2003a: 63–4.

Ayurveda has profoundly influenced all the cultures surrounding South Asia, including Tibet, Central Asia, China, South-East Asia and the Middle East. Through Portuguese and Dutch physicians of the sixteenth and seventeenth centuries, many items of Ayurveda's pharmacopoeia entered European medical knowledge in the Early Modern period. Linnaeus's systematization of the natural world drew heavily on these sources, resulting in the prominent representation of Ayurveda's medicinal legacy in binomial plant taxonomy from the eighteenth century onwards.[3]

Since the mid-nineteenth century, the text of the *Suśrutasaṃhitā* (henceforth *SS*) has been the subject of hundreds of studies, epitomes, commentaries, editions and translations. It has entered the fabric of the history of medicine as one of the best-known Asian medical classics.[4] The *SS* is especially famous for its chapters on surgery, that reveal the extraordinarily advanced methods of plastic surgery, foreign body removal, suturing, cataract removal and other techniques that were known and practiced in classical times.[5] In short, the *SS* is a foundational text in South Asian medical history.

Outline history of the editions

The *SS* was first published in print in the nineteenth-century edition of Madhusudana Gupta.[6] There have been 43 subsequent editions of the work, several partial, and often accompanied by Indian-language translations.[7]

---

[3]Wujastyk 2003b: 406–7.

[4]Meulenbeld 1999–2002 provides a comprehensive survey of research up to 2002; later studies include Wujastyk 2000, Wujastyk 2003a: 61–146, and Valiathan 2007.

[5]Selections are translated and discussed in Wujastyk 2003a: 61–115.

[6]Gupta 1835–1836.

[7]Meulenbeld 1999–2002: IB, 311–14.

The standard vulgate edition of the *SS* is the Bombay edition of Yādavaśarma Trivikrama Ācārya.[8] He based his first edition on three manuscripts (Calcutta, Jaipur, Bundi). In his second edition he added evidence from nine further manuscripts. In the last edition from his hand, the third edition of 1938, he added evidence of three more manuscripts, including one unidentified old palm leaf manuscript in the possession of Hemarājaśarman of Nepal. A diligent and learned editor, Ācārya nevertheless did not use the methods developed in Europe during the Enlightenment and the nineteenth century for evaluating manuscripts and placing their evidence in a structural relationship to each other on the basis of similarities and differences. These methods enable us to make historically-informed judgements about the transmission of the text, i.e., separating *recensio* from *emendatio*. These text-critical methodologies, first developed in forms approaching their modern incarnations by Richard Bentley (1662–1742), Karl Lachmann (1793–1851) and others, were introduced to higher scholarship in India only at the start of the twentieth century, especially through the work of V. S. Sukthankar and his group at the Bhandarkar Oriental Research Institute, the editorial work of D. D. Kosambi on Bhartṛhari's *Śatakatraya*, and the manual of S. M. Katre.[9]

[8] Ācārya 1915.

[9] On the early history of the text-critical method, see Dain 1975, Pasquali 1952, Maas 1958, Timpanaro 2005, Reynolds and Wilson 1991, West 1973, etc. Kosambi's most famous critical edition is his 1948 edition of Bhartṛhari's *Śatakatraya*, although he published several other related editions of the same work, including different commentaries. Sumitra Mangal Katre was the first to author a general introduction to the application of text-critical methods specifically to Indian manuscript materials (Katre 1941). Katre's work was inspired by the application of text-critical methods to the editing of the *Mahābhārata* by his colleague Sukthankar (1933).

Ācārya's goal was common with that of Indian manuscript scribes through the ages: to produce a text that made sense to him and represented what the majority of the manuscripts said.[10] In his footnotes, Ācārya does not normally distinguish between different manuscripts. Variant readings are infrequently noted, normally indiscriminately as "another reading (Skt. *iti pā[ṭhāntaram]*)," alongside selected readings and comments from medieval commentators. Yet, for all its shortcomings, like many vulgates, Ācārya's edition is enormously valuable, and represents what almost all scholars since 1915 have treated as *the* text of this classic work.

The first printed translation of a part of the *Suśrutasaṃhitā* was that of Hessler into Latin, that followed a decade after the *editio princeps*.[11] Apart from numerous translations into Indian languages, Meulenbeld (1999–2002: IB, 314–15) lists eleven translations into non-Indian languages, including one into Japanese, to which can be added the recent translations by Sharma (1999–2001), by Srikantha Murthy (2000–2002), and my own selected translations for Penguin Classics.[12]

The problem

In spite of the importance and deserved fame of the *SS*, there remain fundamental problems about the text that gnaw at the base of all other historical and cultural claims based on it. In the introduction to my own translated section of the *SS*'s chapter "On Breath and Wind," I made the following observations:[13]

---

[10]Colas 1999.

[11]Hessler 1844–1855.

[12]For a survey of early translations of Ayurveda works, see Zysk 1984.

[13]Wujastyk 2003a: 75–6.

> One of the most striking features to the reader of this section of Suśruta's *Compendium* is the poor state of the text. By the time of the commentators Gayadāsa (*ca.* 1000) and Ḍalhaṇa (*ca.* 12th century) many variant readings were in circulation for this part of the text, and these commentators note that the manuscripts available to them had alternative readings to almost every verse. Other parts of Suśruta's *Compendium* are also peppered with uncertain readings, but perhaps not to the same degree as the present chapter. The variability of Suśruta's text was so obvious even a millennium ago that it spurred the creation of a work of medieval textual criticism, Candraṭa's *Suśrutapāṭhaśuddhi*, 'Correction of the readings in Suśruta,' probably written at about the turn of the eleventh century.[14] What all this means for the history of this important text is unclear at present: in the absence of a critical edition and study of the history of the work we can only speculate about the possible causes for this high density of variations.

Although the *SS* holds a position of great importance in the history of medicine, the textual foundations of the work itself are insecure and its interpretation deeply problematic. Meulenbeld has drawn attention to many of these difficulties and to the secondary literature in which scholars have mostly, it must be said, floundered with these questions.[15] Sharma has surveyed the ways in which comment-

[14]Meulenbeld 1974: 409.
[15]Meulenbeld 1999–2002: IA, 336–52.

ators on Sanskrit medical texts can provide important evidence for the history of the texts.[16]

There has never been an attempt at a critical edition of the text, the obvious first step towards addressing these difficulties. Many problems of the history and interpretation of the text are waiting for the application to the *SS* of modern methods of textual criticism and editorial technique, including lower and higher criticism.

The new opportunity

In January 2007, a previously unknown manuscript of the *Suśrutasaṃhitā* was brought to scholarly attention. Dimitrov and Tamot of the Nepalese-German Manuscript Cataloguing Project (NGMCP), based at the University of Hamburg, described the manuscript presently in the Kaiser Shamsher Library, Kathmandu, in the following terms:[17]

> We know about the Licchavi King Mānadeva IV from a very old palm-leaf manuscript of the *Suśrutasaṃhitā*, a medical treatise, which was copied in Deopatan (Gvala) in MS 301 [AD 877] and is now kept in the Kaiser Library (NGMPP, NAK 9/699).

A ninth-century manuscript of the *Suśrutasaṃhitā* is an astonishing discovery for the scientific history of India.

If the manuscript's date holds up to scrutiny, then Kaiser Shamsher NAK 9/699 ranks amongst the earliest manuscripts known from peninsular India. Almost all earlier Indic manuscripts have been found in Northern Pakistan or Central Asia. This manuscript is of far greater importance for the history of science and medicine than

[16] Sharma 2005.

[17] Dimitrov and Tamot 2007: 33.

as a carrier of evidence for a particular Nepalese monarch, however interesting that might be for political history and chronology.

Further investigation in the catalogue of the NGMCP and a preliminary study of images of the manuscript has revealed that Kaiser Shamsher NAK 9/699 is incomplete, though its 127 folios cover about half the *Suśrutasaṃhitā*. The manuscript is written in "Transitional Gupta" script, a particularly archaic form of late medieval North Indian calligraphy that agrees palaeographically with the early date of the colophon. There are three other manuscripts of the *Suśrutasaṃhitā* in the NGMCP's microfilm archive, one dated to the early sixteenth century that appears to be complete. On the grounds of palaeography and other codicological factors, it is safe to assert that all three of these other manuscripts are relatively early, and certainly important for the history of the text.[18]

The discovery of this new, early manuscript for part of the *Suśrutasaṃhitā* brings a new focus and urgency to the problem. For the first time, we have textual evidence that potentially takes our knowledge of this work back *a thousand years* earlier than any previously known evidence. It is important, to say the least, to evaluate this new evidence, and to attempt to clarify the textual history of the *Suśrutasaṃhitā*.

Amongst many interesting questions that the study of this manuscript would allow one to address, Meulenbeld has noted that a ninth-century *Suśrutasaṃhitā* manuscript would enable us to examine whether or not the learned medical historian Prof. P. V. Sharma was right in his asser-

[18]The Kaiser Shamsher National Archives of Kathmandu accession numbers for these manuscripts are 9/699, 5/333, 5/334 and 1/1146.

tion that the vulgate text represents a version updated by the tenth-century author Candraṭa.[19]

A preliminary examination of Kaiser Shamsher NAK 9/699 has already revealed a startling fact. It frequently lacks the standard phrase *yathovāca bhagavān dhanvantariḥ* "as the sage Dhanvantari declared," that appears at the start of all chapters in the vulgate text.[20] This phrase casts the entire work as a series of lectures made by the ancient sage Dhanvantari. This basic change to the text entirely re-frames the work, and throws into question the standard traditional accounts of the origin of the work. Furthermore, preliminary consultation with the Vienna *Carakasaṃhitā* project suggests that some of the *Carakasaṃhitā* manuscripts collected by that project also lack the parallel framing *Ātreya* narrative that is associated with the Caraka text.[21] This points to the possible existence of a critically important editorial moment in the history of these texts, perhaps in the tenth century, when they were re-framed to fit a particular narrative of origin.[22]

The wider manuscript base

Although the discovery of this thousand-year old manuscript and its companions in Kathmandu is exciting and likely to be of great importance for the study of the text, "manuscripts should be weighed, not counted".[23] At a rough estimate, there may be as many as two hundred

[19]Personal communication. For more detail on this view, see Meulenbeld 1999–2002: IA, 341. Sharma's view is given in his publications of 1975: 66–67 and 1992: 200–201.

[20]See now, e.g., for the omitted phrase *yathovāca bhagavān dhanvantariḥ* in Klebanov 2010: p.83, n. 5 *ad* Su.śl.4.1, and p. 86, n. 1, *ad* Su.śl.15.1.

[21]Prof. Dr Karin Preisendanz, personal communication.

[22]Cf. the study by Zysk 1999.

[23]West 1973: 49.

manuscripts of the *Suśrutasaṃhitā* in existence in libraries worldwide.[24] Many, if not most, of these are fragmentary or partial. Nevertheless, it is important to study previously unexamined manuscript evidence for the portion of the text covered by Kaiser Shamsher NAK 9/699.

As West so wisely noted,[25]

> Of the whole collating project, the hardest part to carry out with complete success is probably the business of finding out what manuscripts there are.

The starting point for tracking down Indian manuscripts is always Aufrecht's *Catalogus Catalogorum* (1891–1903), but this work now represents only a fraction of the manuscript wealth that has come to light during the last century. The University of Madras has been running a project since 1968 to update Aufrecht's work and to publish a unified census of Sanskrit manuscripts from catalogued library collections worldwide. The portion of the *New Catalogus Catalogorum* that would cover the *Suśrutasaṃhitā* manuscripts is still several years away from publication, although the publication rate of the project rate has recently accelerated greatly with the publication of five new volumes in 2008. Nevertheless, consultation with the project staff and the unpublished files of the project remains a necessity.[26] This information can form a valuable aid for planning a manuscript photographing campaign.

Field experience in conducting manuscript searches in India gives one no illusions about the rates of success in actually getting photographs of the manuscripts one needs.

[24]Biswas and Prajapati (1998) provide the most up-to-date published listing of catalogued Sanskrit manuscript collections.

[25]West 1973: 64.

[26]Raghavan *et al.* 1949–.

But Indian manuscripts are many and librarians are often hospitable and helpful. With tact and patience, much can be achieved in spite of the difficulties. It seems reasonable to believe that a substantial number of manuscripts of the *Suśrutasaṃhitā* could be photographed in a reasonable time. In any case, we can comfort ourselves with "Kosambi's Law of Manuscripts," that predicts that the manuscripts that can be accessed most readily for scholarly purposes are likely to include the most important textual witnesses.[27]

Research methods

Combining the textual evidence from a number of previously unexamined manuscripts with the evidence of the new Kaiser Shamsher NAK 9/699 makes possible a fresh edition of a meaningful portion of the *Suśrutasaṃhitā*. It also makes possible the arrangement of manuscripts into groups or families. Indian manuscripts (like Greek and Latin ones) are normally horizontally contaminated by scribal comparisons. While a *stemma codicum* of the type analysed by Paul Maas (1958) is normally impossible with contaminated transmissions, a great deal of understanding and clarification of the text can come from grouping manuscripts into meaningful families.

Collation

The four newly-discovered manuscripts from Nepal need to be collated against the vulgate edition of Ācārya, unless they depart from the text so radically that it becomes pointless to proceed. In that case, a diplomatic transcription of Kaiser Shamsher NAK 9/699 can form the basis for further

[27]Kosambi 1948: 10: "It is a general rule (Kosambi's law!) that the actual use-value of a MS is inversely proportional to the fuss made in lending it."

collation. This work on the Nepalese manuscripts requires skills in reading Transitional Gupta script.

Survey of MSS

A survey of discoverable manuscripts of the *Suśrutasaṃhitā* needs to be developed in consultation with the *New Catalogus Catalogorum* project in Chennai, the Indira Gandhi National Centre for the Arts (IGNCA) in Delhi and the National Mission for Manuscripts (NAMAMI), also in Delhi. The IGNCA has very large holdings of microfilmed Sanskrit manuscripts, including medical materials, and is likely to have several *Suśrutasaṃhitā* manuscripts microfilmed in its collection.

The focus of the research as outlined here is on evaluating the new textual data from Kaiser Shamsher NAK 9/699 and the accompanying Nepalese MSS. However, the data of the other Nepalese manuscripts is likely to be of similar importance and their inclusion may enable a full, continuous "Nepalese" text of the *SS* to be edited.

A survey of *Suśrutasaṃhitā* manuscripts from all other known repositories would, in itself, be a most valuable research tool.[28]

Manuscript evaluation

Once a reasonably comprehensive list of existing *Suśrutasaṃhitā* manuscripts has been developed, and some have been acquired in microfilm or digitally, the work of weighing them can be undertaken. This is carried out by spot-collating a small number of relatively short passages from various parts of the work. This work has a specific goal, namely to establish, as far as possible, relationships

[28]The value of this type of codicological research is discussed in Wujastyk 2008.

between the manuscripts, and especially to discover any manuscripts that might belong with NAK 9/699 as early witnesses to the text of the *Suśrutasaṃhitā*.

The processes of manuscript evaluation can be extended at a subsequent stage of work into a full stemmatic analysis, as exemplified by the work done by the members of the University of Vienna's Caraka Project on the manuscript tradition of the *Carakasaṃhitā*.[29]

Fieldwork

Visits to manuscript libraries in India and Nepal, and resource-centres such as the IGNCA in New Delhi, afford the opportunity of examining, photographing and/or collating *Suśrutasaṃhitā* manuscripts at the Kaiser Shamsher and other repositories. Collections where *Suśrutasaṃhitā* MSS are already known to exist include the Bhandarkar Institute (Pune, 5 partial MSS), the Rajasthan Oriental Research Institute (Jodhpur), the Sarasvati Bhavan (Varanasi), the DAV College (Chandigarh), and the Government Oriental Manuscripts Library (Chennai, one partial MS). These are all major libraries, but none of their collections are fully catalogued, and personal visits are necessary. In general, for historical and textual reasons beyond the scope of this report, it is to be expected that *Suśrutasaṃhitā* manuscripts may be more commonly found in north Indian collections than elsewhere.

---

[29]On the Caraka Project, see `http://www.istb.univie.ac.at/caraka`. Publications on the stemmatic analysis of Sanskrit medical texts include those in the present volume, as well as Maas 2010a,b, and Pecchia 2010.

Conclusion

The appearance of new manuscript information through the labours of the Nepal-German Manuscript Cataloguing Project has been quietly revolutionizing many fields of premodern Indian literature, including especially *purāṇa* and *tantra* literature. Now, the discovery of a thousand-year old medical manuscript of the *SS* offers us the opportunity to develop a new and more secure understanding of the history and meaning of Suśruta's medical classic. The steps towards this goal have been outlined, and illustrate the procedures necessary to make progress with finding, evaluating and editing Sanskrit scientific manuscripts.

Epilogue

After the first version of this paper was written, and partly inspired by it (Klebanov 2010: 60), Andrey Klebanov took up the study of MS NAK 9/699 as a thesis project for the master's degree at the University of Hamburg.[30] The results are a very promising beginning in the critical study of this unique manuscript, and the manuscript group with which it has been preserved.

References

Ācārya, Yādavaśarman Trivikrama (ed.) 1915. *Suśrutasaṃhitā, Suśrutena viracitā, Vaidyavaraśrīḍalhaṇācāryaviracitayā Nibandhasaṃgrahākhyavyākhyayā samullasitā, Ācāryopāhvena Trivikramātmajena Yādavaśarmaṇṇā saṃśodhitā*. Mumbayyāṃ: Nirṇayasāgara Mudrāyantrālaye.

Aufrecht, Th. 1891–1903. *Catalogus Catalogorum, an Alphabetical Register of Works and Authors*. Leipzig: German Oriental Society.

[30] Klebanov 2010.

Biswas, Subhas C. and M. K. Prajapati 1998. *Bibliographic Survey of Indian Manuscript Catalogues: Being a Union List of Manuscript Catalogues*. Delhi: Eastern Book Linkers.

Colas, Gérard 1999. "The Criticism and Transmission of Texts in Classical India." *Diogenes*, **47(2)**, 30–43.

Dain, A. 1975. *Les Manuscrits*. Collection d'Études Anciennes Publié sou le patronage d l'Association Guillaume Budé. Paris: Société d'Édition "Les Belles-Lettres", 3rd edn. First published, 1949.

Dimitrov, Dragomir and Kashinath Tamot 2007. "Kaiser Shamsher, his Library and his Manuscript Collection." *Newsletter of the NGMCP [Nepal-German Manuscript Cataloguing Project]*, **3**, 26–36. `http://www.uni-hamburg.de/ngmcp/newsletter.html`.

Gupta, Sri Madhusudana (ed.) 1835–1836. *Āyur-veda-prakāśa [also called Suśruta-saṃhitā] by Suśruta. The Suśruta, or System of Medicine, Taught by Dhanwantari, and Composed by his Disciple Suśruta*. Calcutta: Education Press and Baptist Mission Press.

Hessler, Franz 1844–1855. *Ayurvédas: id est medicinae systema a venerabili D'Hanvantare demonstratum a Susruta discipulo compositum; Nunc primum ex Sanskrita in Latinum sermonem vertit, introductionem, annotationes et rerum indice Franciscus Hessler*. Erlangen: Ferdinandum Enke. 3v.

Katre, S. M. 1941. *Introduction to Indian Textual Criticism*. Bombay: Karnatak Publishing House. With appendix II, "A Brief Note on the History and Progress of Cataloguing of Sanskrit and other MSS in India and Outside (between AD 1800 and 1941)" by P. K. Gode.

Klebanov, Andrey 2010. *The *Nepalese Version of the Suśruta-saṃhitā and its Interrelation with Buddhism and the Buddhists*. MA thesis, Hamburg University, Hamburg.

Kosambi, D. D. 1948. *Bhartṛhari-Viracitaḥ Śatakatrayādi-Subhāṣitasaṃgrahaḥ. Mahākavi-Bhartṛharipraṇītatvena Nīti-*

Śṛṅgāra-Vairāgyādināmnā samākhyātānāṃ Subhāṣitānāṃ Supariṣkṛtasaṃgrahaḥ) Suvistṛtaparicayātmikyāṅglaprastāvanā-vividhapāṭhāntara-pariśiṣṭādisamanvitaḥ ācāryaśrīJinavijayālekhitāgravacanālaṃkṛtaś ca = The Epigrams Attributed to Bhartṛhari. Including the Three Centuries for the First Time Collected and Critically Edited, with Principal Variants and an Introduction, vol. 23 of *Singhi Jain Series*. Baṃbaī: Bhāratīya Vidyā Bhavana, 1st edn.

Maas, Paul 1958. *Textual Criticism. Translated from the German by Barbara Flower*. Oxford: Clarendon Press.

Maas, Philipp A. 2010a. "Computer Aided Stemmatics – The Case of Fifty-Two Text Versions of Carakasaṃhitā Vimānasthāna 8.67–157." *Wiener Zeitschrift für die Kunde Südasiens*, **52–53**, 63–119.

— 2010b. "On What Became of the Carakasaṃhitā After Dṛḍhabala's Revision." *eJournal of Indian Medicine*, **3**, 1–22.

Meulenbeld, Gerrit Jan 1974. *The Mādhavanidāna and its Chief Commentary: Chapters 1–10. Introduction, Translation, and Notes*. Leiden: Brill.

— 1999–2002. *A History of Indian Medical Literature*, vol. XV of *Groningen Oriental Studies*. Groningen: E. Forsten. 5v.

Pasquali, Giorgio 1952. *Storia della tradizione e critica del testo*. Firenze: Felice le Monnier, 2nd edn. 1st ed. 1934.

Pecchia, Cristina 2010. "Transmission-specific (In)utility, or Dealing with Contamination: Samples from the Textual Tradition of the Carakasaṃhitā." *Wiener Zeitschrift für die Kunde Südasiens*, **52–53**, 121–59.

Raghavan, V., K. Kunjunni Raja, C. S. Sundaram, N. Veezhinathan, N. Gangadharan, *et al.* 1949–. *New Catalogus Catalogorum, an Alphabetical Register of Sanskrit and Allied Works and Authors*. Madras University Sanskrit Series. Madras: University of Madras.

Reynolds, Leighton D. and Nigel G. Wilson 1991. *Scribes*

and Scholars. A Guide to the Transmission of Greek and Latin Literature. Oxford: Clarendon Press, 3rd edn. 1st ed. 1968.

Sharma, Priya Vrat 1975. *Āyurved kā Vaijñānik Itihās*, vol. 1 of *Jayakṛṣṇadāsa Āyurveda Granthamālā*. Vārāṇasī: Caukhambā Orientalia. Reference is to the 2004 reprint.

Sharma, Priya Vrat (ed.) 1992. *History of Medicine in India*. New Delhi: Indian National Science Academy.

Sharma, Priya Vrat 1999–2001. *Suśruta-Saṃhitā, with English Translation of Text and Ḍalhaṇa's Commentary Alongwith* (sic) *Critical Notes*, vol. 9 of *Haridas Ayurveda Series*. Varanasi: Chaukhambha Visvabharati. 3v.

— 2005. "Role of Commentators in Textual Criticism." In Satya Deo Dubey and Anugrah Narain Singh (eds.), *Six Decades of Ayurveda (1941–2000): A Collection of the Selected Articles and Lectures by Prof. Priya Vrat Sharma*, vol. 37 of *The Vrajajiwan Ayurvijnan Granthamala*, chap. 11, pp. 114–26. Delhi: Chaukhamba Sanskrit Pratishthan.

Srikantha Murthy, K. R. 2000–2002. *Illustrated Suśruta saṃhitā: Text, English Translation, Notes, Appendices and Index*, vol. 102 of *Jaikrishnadas Ayurveda Series*. Varanasi: Chaukhambha Orientalia. 3v.

Sukthankar, S. Vishnu 1933. "Prolegomena." In S[itaram] Vishnu Sukthankar, S[hripad] K[rishna] Belvalkar, *et al.* (eds.), *The Ādiparvan, being the First Book of the Mahābhārata, the Great Epic of India*, pp. i–cx. Poona: Bhandarkar Oriental Research Institute.

Timpanaro, Sebastiano 2005. *The Genesis of Lachmann's Method, Edited and Translated [from Italian into English] by Glenn W. Most*. Chicago and London: University of Chicago Press. Original Italian edition, *La genesi del metodo del Lachmann*, Padova 1971.

Valiathan, M. S. 2007. *The Legacy of Suśruta*. Hyderabad, Chennai, etc.: Orient Longman.

Vogel, Claus 1981. "On Editing Indian Codices Unici (With

Special Reference to the Gilgit Manuscripts)." In H. von Stietencron (ed.), *Indology in India and Germany: Problems of Information, Coordination and Cooperation*, pp. 59–69. Tübingen: Seminar für Indologie und Vergleichende Religionswissenschaft.

West, Martin L. 1973. *Textual Criticism and Editorial Technique applicable to Greek and Latin Texts*. Stuttgart: Teubner.

Wujastyk, Dominik 2000. "The Combinatorics of Tastes and Humours in Classical Indian Medicine and Mathematics." *Journal of Indian Philosophy*, **28**, 479–95.

— 2003a. *The Roots of Āyurveda: Selections from Sanskrit Medical Writings*. London, New York, etc.: Penguin Group, 3rd edn.

— 2003b. "The Science of Medicine." In Gavin Flood (ed.), *The Blackwell Companion to Hinduism*, chap. 19, pp. 393–409. Oxford: Blackwell.

— 2008. "A Pilot Census of the Medical Sciences in Sanskrit." *Journal of the Indian Institute of History of Medicine*, **38**, 111–56.

Zysk, Kenneth G. 1984. "An Annoted Bibliography of Translations into Western Languages of Principle Sanskrit Medical Treatises." *Clio Medica*, **19(3–4)**, 281–91.

— 1991. *Asceticism and Healing in Ancient India: Medicine in the Buddhist Monastery*. New York, Bombay, etc.: Oxford University Press. Reprinted, Delhi 1998 and 2000.

— 1999. "Mythology and the Brāhmaṇization of Indian Medicine: Transforming Heterodoxy into Orthodoxy." In Folke Josephson (ed.), *Categorisation and Interpretation*, pp. 125–45. Göteborg: Meijerbergs institut för svensk etymologisk forskning, Göteborgs universitet.

5

Anthony Cerulli

The Joy of Life: Medicine, Politics, and Religion

In the long history of Sanskrit literature, storytelling is a common means of instruction and argument. Although it is by no means ubiquitous in Sanskrit medical literature, there are some remarkable narratives about bodily well-being in Ayurvedic literature. Recent scholarship on Indian medical history has frequently disregarded these narratives. If scholars addressed these narratives, they have tended to explain them away as remnants of an old tension between practitioners of classical medicine and religion.[1] Medical themes embedded in narrative texts include the etiologies of fever (in the myth of Dakṣa's sacrifice), miscarriage (in the story of Revatī's *avatāra* Jātahāriṇī), and tuberculosis (in the myth of the "king's disease," *rājayakṣman*). These are just a few of the more well known narratives in the classical

I would like to thank Dr. P. Ram Manohar and the Arya Vaidya Pharmacy in Coimbatore, Tamilnadu for inviting me to present an earlier draft of this paper. I also thank CATS and its members for their ongoing and excellent work on the history of Indian medicine and Sanskrit medical literature.

[1]See, for example, Chattopadhyaya 1986, Zysk 1991: 118, Thapar 2002: 258, Engler 2003: 233–36 *et passim*.

medical compendia of Caraka, Suśruta, Vāgbhaṭa, Bhela, and Kaśyapa.[2] Narrative instruction, however, is rather atypical in these medical works, which by and large convey a rigorously positivistic science shorn of dramatic flair. Several centuries after the classical period, around the turn of the 17th-18th centuries in Thanjavur, South India, during the reign of King Śāhaji (1684–1712)[3], Ānandarāyamakhin (hereafter Ānandarāya) produced a remarkable Sanskrit allegory, *The Joy of Life* (*Jīvānandanam*), which uses drama as the primary vehicle for imparting medical knowledge. Ānandarāya's use of a sustained allegorical narrative to express Ayurvedic principles is innovative in the history of Indian medical literature. He presents a nuanced and complex picture of cultural discourse and social construction in the story, which ultimately makes *The Joy of Life* a useful starting point for rethinking methodological approaches to the study of Ayurveda and the contribution of Indian medical discourse to Indian cultural history. In this chapter, I present a portion of the groundwork from my work on an English translation of *The Joy of Life*. I pay special attention to the discursive interplay of medicine, statecraft, and religion in the text. Ānandarāya deftly used these three knowledge systems in his play to articulate an expansive notion of well-being that interweaves and co-implicates the individual person and society. To conclude, I offer an act-by-act synopsis of the play.

There are four edited Sanskrit editions of *The Joy of Life*:

1881, Mysore edited by Vyasacharya.

[2] I treat these three medical narratives at length, in terms of their literary history and medical functions, in Cerulli 2007.

[3] Heinrich Zimmer mistakenly assigned the date of the *Jīvānandanam* (which he translated as "The Bliss of the Life-Monad or Soul") to the first half of the seventeenth century (Zimmer 1979: 61).

1891, Mumbai	edited by Dvivedī and Paraba.
1933, Khurja	edited by Nārāyaṇadatta.
1947, Madras	edited by Duraisvāmi Ayyaṅgār.

To date, there have been only two translations of *The Joy of Life*, both of which are in European languages:

1929, Italian	translated by Vallauri.
1937, German	translated by Weckerling.

There are no translations of the play in a South Asian language.

Context, authorship, and contribution

At the outset of the play, the stage manager (*sūtradhāraḥ*) explains that *The Joy of Life* was composed for live performance at the Bṛhadīśvara Temple Festival in Thanjavur, Tamil Nadu. His remarks establish the historical and authorial information for the dramatic performance to follow:

Stage Manager: Listen! Here in the city of Thanjavur, country and city folk from many places have come together hoping to see the chariot festival of Maheśvara (Śiva). These members of the assembly have become touchstones to discern the gold that is called poetry that moves the heart. They are receptacles of priceless judgment and playgrounds for the Six Darśanas. They are rewards for my austerities, and they have made me eager. My heart wants to honor them here with this play.

Asst. Stage Manager (shaking his head):
On what will the composition be based?

Stage Manager: Well, I am producing a new play called "The Joy of Life."

Asst. Stage Manager:
Who wrote the script?

Stage Manager: Ānandarāyamakhin. He is the wish-granting tree of the learned poets.[4]

It is evident straight away that Ānandarāya's play was intended for mass consumption, apparently to educate and entertain the public through drama. This fact alone sets Ānandarāya's work apart from other Sanskrit works in the history of Indian medicine, for *The Joy of Life* is the only existing piece of Sanskrit medical literature that was clearly composed for this purpose. That Ānandarāya declares the play to be a performance piece, and that the play's content has clear medical significance, suggest that the practice of narrativizing the body for medical purposes has been known for at least three centuries in South Asian history. A thorough study of *The Joy of Life* is thus an important step in the development of our understanding of how medical

---

[4] *Jīvānandanam* 1.5ff. (Duraisvāmi Ayyaṅgār 1947: 6–8):
Sūtradhāraḥ: śṛṇu tāvat. atra tañjāpure paurajānapadā deśāntarād āgatāś ca bṛhadīśvararathotsavadidṛkṣayā saṅghībhūtāḥ

sarasakavitānāmno hemnaḥ kaṣopalatāṃ gatāḥ
viharaṇabhuvaḥ ṣaḍdarśinyā vivekadhanākarāḥ|
vidadhati tapolabhyāḥ sabhyā ime mama kautukaṃ
tad iha hṛdayaṃ nāṭyenaitān upāsitum īhate|| 5 ||

Pāripārśvakaḥ: (saśiraḥkampam) kaṃ punaḥ prabandham avalambya?
Sūtradhāraḥ: nanv asti mama vaśe jīvānandanaṃ nāma navīnaṃ nāṭakam.
Pāripārśvakaḥ: kas tasya prabandhasya kaviḥ?
Sūtradhāraḥ: vidvatkavikalpataruḥ ānandarāyamakhī.

narrative has functioned in South Asia, and indeed how it continues to function today in forms such as street theatre and some traditional clinical practice.

The Joy of Life unfolds simultaneously inside and outside the body of the play's hero, King Life (*Jīvarāja*). The play's characters concurrently represent parts of the human body and actors in a royal society. The basic idea of the allegory is that the physiology of the human body affects, communicates with, and is under the influence of the social physiology of its surroundings. The result is a collision of physiologies, so to speak. In terms of the narrative, King Life must learn how to reconcile his own welfare with the events of the often-deleterious world around him. In particular, King Life is confronted with an attack by the dreadful personification of *rājayakṣman*, King Disease.

At the symbolic level, I read Ānandarāya's depiction of King Life and the paths he takes to thwart King Disease's assault as a commentary on the opposing principles of outward-focussed action and inward-focussed action (*pravṛtti* and *nivṛtti*) in classical Indian philosophy.[5] As I discuss below, political governance and religion, or more precisely royal statecraft and ascetic withdrawal from the world, correspondingly characterize these two types of action in *The Joy of Life*. The chief medical assertion of the play, I contend, is that the commitment to the health, or well-being, of one's body (what I have called one's "body-dharma" elsewhere) is a fundamental human obligation as well as a necessary prerequisite to enable the pursuit of both activity in the world (*pravṛtti*) and religious practice involving a degree of worldly withdrawal (*nivṛtti*).[6]

[5]On *pravṛtti/nivṛtti*, see, e.g., Bailey 1985.

[6]Cerulli 2007.

Over the course of the last century, there has been some debate about the purported author of *The Joy of Life*. A handful of scholars have endorsed someone named Vedakavi as the author of the play.[7] Proponents of this endorsement have on the whole neglected to explain why the text should be ascribed to Vedakavi rather than Ānandarāya. Apparently following the lead of Kuppuswamy Sastri (1904), who was the first to make the unsubstantiated assertion of Vedakavi's authorship, the argument is that Ānandarāya was Vedakavi's patron. The text itself neither explicitly supports this argument nor, for that matter, does it once mention the name Vedakavi. Rather, the text says the play was written by Ānandarāya (*jīvānandanam Ānandarāyamakhinā praṇītaṃ*).[8] To suggest that this acknowledgement of authorship is simply honorary or representative is to my mind unwarranted. The advocates of Vedakavi as the play's author have suggested the same argument concerning another allegory attributed to Ānandarāya, *The Nuptials of Knowledge* (*Vidyāpariṇayam*).[9] For the sake of brevity and consistency, I do not take up this debate here. Instead, I follow the text and proceed on the statement of the text itself as though Ānandarāya, not Vedakavi, wrote *The Joy of Life*.

Who, then, was Ānandarāya? And what are the fundamental contributions of *The Joy of Life* to our existing knowledge of Sanskrit allegory and medical literature?

---

[7]Kuppuswamy Sastri 1904: 181, Subramanian 1928: 32–33, Raghavan 1952: 29, Shekhar 1960: 172, n. 7, and Meulenbeld 1999–2002: IIA, 345.

[8]See also Duraisvāmi Ayyaṅgār 1947: 8–9, ślokas 6–7. Unless otherwise noted, I use Duraisvāmi Ayyaṅgār's edition of the *Jīvānandanam*.

[9]Edited by Rāmā (1991). There is a lot of character overlap between the *Vidyāpariṇayam* and the *Jīvānandanam*. But while the *Jīvānandanam* focuses on medicine, statecraft, and religious devotionalism, the *Vidyāpariṇayam* focuses on Advaita Vedānta philosophy.

In the text itself, we learn that Ānandarāya came from a family of gifted writers, artists, and court officials. In the Thanjavur court of Śāhaji II, as Heinrich Zimmer noted, Ānandarāya was a veritable factotum, "at once chancellor, house-priest, spiritual advisor and court poet".[10] The two works normally ascribed to him, *The Joy of Life* and *The Nuptials of Knowledge*, are both allegories. Based on the allegorical style and structure of both of these works, it appears that Ānandarāya drew inspiration from and deliberately modelled his own allegories on Kṛṣṇamiśra's *Prabodhacandrodaya* and Vedānta Deśika's *Saṃkalpasūryodaya*.[11]

Ānandarāya draws together three important Indian knowledge-systems in *The Joy of Life*: government and diplomacy (*arthaśāstra*), religious devotionalism (*bhakti*), and medicine (*āyurveda*). Each one of these themes is expressed in the text through direct quotations from important Sanskrit works in each field, such as Arthaśāstra, *Bhagavadgītā* and the Purāṇas, and Ayurveda. In the introduction to

[10]Zimmer 1979: 61–62.

[11]See, for example, Duraisvāmi Ayyaṅgār's commentary on the *Jīvānandanam* (1947: xii). Kṛṣṇamiśra and Vedānta Deśika were of course not the first people to use allegorical techniques in Sanskrit literature. Although, as Shekhar observed, the *Prabodhacandrodaya* is the earliest known sustained allegorical drama in Sanskrit: "Whatever be the actual state of affairs [before the *Prabodhacandrodaya*, ca., mid to late 11th century CE] the credit of composing the first allegorical play goes to Kṛṣṇamiśra" (Shekhar 1960: 194). Before Kṛṣṇamiśra, fragments from Aśvaghoṣa reveal the use of allegorical techniques, most notably in his three characters Fame (*Kīrti*), Firmness (*Dhṛti*), and Wisdom (*Buddhi*). After Aśvaghoṣa, in the 9th century C.E., Jayanta Bhaṭṭa (author of the *Nyāyamañjari*) wrote a highly didactic and philosophical play, the *Āgamaḍambara*, that contains shades of allegorical ornamentation (Nambiar 1998: 2). Following Kṛṣṇamiśra's *Prabodhacandrodaya*, numerous Sanskrit allegories were composed, such as Yaśapāla's *Mohaparājaya* and Karṇapūra's *Caitanyacandrodaya* (Shekhar 1960: 195).

his German translation of the play, Adolf Weckerling argued that the basic ideology of *The Joy of Life* is religion, particularly Śaiva devotionalism.[12] More recently, Maria Schetelich has suggested that Ānandarāya's play is primarily a meditation on civic authority and leadership.[13] Mario Vallauri highlighted the breadth of Ānandarāya's interests in his Italian translation of the play. Among the themes he identified, the most central are medicine, myth and religion, philosophy, politics, and poetics.[14] There is a single unifying theme in *The Joy of Life* upon which all other subjects hang, however, and that theme is medicine (Ayurveda). In particular, Ānandarāya's play relates a message about how best to superintend the physical body so that it functions in the world of objects in its most optimal ways. The themes of statecraft and religion are indeed present in the play. But the theme of religious devotion supports, rather than guides, the elaboration of the play's numerous medical and somatic lessons. The theme of statecraft represents the duty (*dharma*) of the play's hero, King Life, to which he must attend; but it is a secondary obligation to be pursued after he cares for his body, the cultivation of which is his primary duty.[15]

Sorting through the themes

Over seven equally poetic, scientific, and at time bawdy acts, *The Joy of Life* demonstrates that Ayurvedic medicine is a fine art of adjusting the body's parts and immuno-

[12] Weckerling 1937: 36-38.

[13] Schetelich 1984: 299-330, esp. 300-302.

[14] Vallauri 1929: vii-xiv.

[15] Meulenbeld 1999–2002: 345–46. Again, in a forthcoming article, I treat the notion of "body-dharma" in Ayurveda at length in Sanskrit medical literature apart from the *Joy of Life*. Ānandarāya's play is in many ways the paradigmatic illustration of the body-dharma concept.

defenses to support the demands of a person's social relationships and religious duties. In the play, King Life has a clear responsibility to care for his body. This is, so to speak, his body-dharma. The ways in which King Life attends to this dharma serves as the play's model to address how the human body responds to disease and how the body may be improved so that a person can effectively carry out his or her religious dharmas (such as, the dharma of class and stage of life, Sanskrit *varṇa* and *āśrama*).

Ānandarāya's choice of the king as the model of body dharma is significant. In the ancient Indian context many people relied on the king for protection and sustenance, and if the king went down he took many people with him. But the king in *The Joy of Life* mustn't be read merely as a royal sovereign of subjects and territories, which inevitably occludes a personal identification of the play's audience with the play's hero. Instead, the allegorical nature of King Life symbolizes self-sovereignty, the person who is a king unto himself (or queen unto herself). Simply put, King Life is a human being. The various predicaments in which he finds himself in Ānandarāya's play collectively form a fundamental question that arises from being human, a question with which most people at some point in their lives are confronted. That question is: How do I superintend my physical body in the face of illness, mental unrest, and religious uncertainty? In this way, the basic message of Ānandarāya's play has the capacity to resonate with diverse groups of people. That the play employs warfare terminology and imagery to describe immunological details to a general audience moreover signals a utilitarian, state-managed approach to maintain the health of the body politic. The use of military metaphors to explain disease pathology and treatment often reflects concerns and anxieties not only about individual bodily health, but also about wider rifts, concerns, and unease in society. Writing about the use of military imagery in medical discourse, Deborah Lupton has commented that "while military imagery may overtly connote decisive action and the refusal to 'give in' to the disease, at a deeper level of meaning this discourse serves to draw boundaries between Self and Other by representing the body as a nation state which is vulnerable to attacks by foreign invaders, invoking and resolving anxieties to do with xenophobia, invasion, control and contamination".[16] Military imagery in *The Joy of Life* links illness – indeed even just the threat of illness – to politics, religion, war, fear, violence, control, and heroism. In so doing, Ānandarāya situates medical discourse squarely in the middle of common cultural categories and emotional states that would have made the medical issues in his play highly relevant to an audience of nonmedical practitioners.[17]

The Joy of Life in effect reiterates what the classical Sanskrit medical sources established centuries earlier: Ayurvedic knowledge offers both empirical and normative information about how to make the human body healthy in order to attend to other duties, or *dharma*s, in one's lifetime. To maintain a state of physical health King Life must come to terms with, and ultimately accept, his dharma as a warrior-king (*kṣatriya*). At the same time he makes a great effort to integrate religious devotionalism (*bhakti*) within his Kṣatriya dharma. With the presentation of this balancing act, Ānandarāya works with a common motif in Sanskrit literature. For example, the question about whether or not to act in line with one's own dharma evokes the well-known and fundamental problem of the *Bhaga*-

[16]Lupton 2003: 69.

[17]Lupton 2003: 83.

vadgītā when the Pāṇḍava warrior Arjuna considers sitting out of the impending battle with his cousins, the Kauravas. Arjuna receives guidance from Kṛṣṇa, whose advice to the wavering warrior is far from straightforward, and his teachings in the *Gītā* have been interpreted in many, often conflicting ways. All the same, many modern commentators on the *Gītā* identify Kṛṣṇa's charge to Arjuna to follow the dharma of his Kṣatriya class as utterly fundamental to Kṛṣṇa's instruction. In Book Two, Kṛṣṇa exclaims: "Look only to your own dharma. Do not quiver before it ..."[18] King Life's reaction to the attack of King Disease's army in *The Joy of Life* in many ways echoes Arjuna's indecision in the *Bhagavadgītā*. Throughout much of Ānandarāya's play King Life cannot decide if he should be engaged in the world as a Kṣatriya king's dharma necessitates or if he should withdraw from the world into a life of ascetic contemplation. A central problem for Arjuna in the *Bhagavadgītā* as well as for King Life in *The Joy of Life* has to do with each individual's understanding of his position and function in the grand scheme of Hindu cosmology.

To discern his place in the universal scheme of things, King Life weighs the recommendations of his two primary advisors, Worldly Knowledge (*Vijñānaśarman*) and Higher Knowledge (*Jñānaśarman*), who separately symbolize, and thus advise King Life to take, the paths of outward-focussed action (*pravṛtti*) and inward-focussed action (*nivṛtti*), respectively. Worldly Knowledge advises King Life on matters pertaining to the first three of the four goals of human life (*puruṣārthas*), or what in *The Joy of Life* and in Sanskrit medical literature are often called the "three things" (*trivarga*): socio-religious duty (Sanskrit *dharma*), material

[18] *Bhagavadgītā* 2:31 (Sastry 2001): *svadharmaṃ cāvekṣya na vikampitum arhasi* ....

prosperity (*artha*), and sexual satisfaction (*kāma*). Conversely, Higher Knowledge advises King Life on matters pertaining to the fourth goal of human life, release (*mokṣa*) from the worldly cycle of rebirth and redeath (*saṃsāra*). King Life's two advisors press him towards their respective priorities throughout the play, while simultaneously trying to persuade the king to reject the advice of the other advisor. Early on, King Life heeds the advice of Higher Knowledge; thus he devotes the bulk of his energies to transcendental matters of the mind and self. But, as Maria Schetelich has observed, Worldly Knowledge's rational and grounded way of thinking swiftly becomes vital to King Life's well-being because military and political strategies are needed to keep his body intact against King Disease's assault.[19]

The importance of religion in the play, specifically Hindu dharma and devotional Śaivism, to the maintenance of bodily health is critical. Religious practice leads King Life to realize perfectly his function on earth as king, that is, to realize his royal dharma (Skt. *rājadharma*). This realization is heavy indeed, for King Life learns that the dharmic obligations of kings are endless and immense. Ānandarāya employs Worldly Knowledge to describe King Life's dharma, which involves an array of outward-looking, diplomatic actions. To paraphrase the text, by granting favours to old Brahmins who have performed difficult religious austerities and by regularly giving gifts to those worthy of donations for their prior devotion, the king protects himself. After establishing his authority over the surface of the earth, the king must govern the whole kingdom. By following the path of dharma, the king resolves to protect his subjects thoroughly. In short, every consideration

[19]Schetelich 1984: 300, n. 7.

the king must make is always for the sake of prosperity for his advisors and friends, kingdom, treasury and housing, and military.[20]

This description of the king's dharma is in line with the concept of outward-focussed action (*pravṛtti*) allegorized in the play by the advisor Worldly Knowledge. The message echoes Kṛṣṇa's injunction to Arjuna in the *Gītā* that the Kṣatriya king must not retreat from battle. For the king is a social lynchpin, the most vital actor in premodern Indian society, and his governing principle is his dharma. King Life's own safety and bodily well-being, Worldly Knowledge explains, should be his primary interest, and he should ensure it by conciliating the important religious figures in his court with gifts; this charity ultimately solidifies the religious authorities' loyalty to the king. With the support of the religious leaders, the king should then turn his attention to the cultivation of happiness and prosperity (literally "a better tomorrow," *śvaḥśreyasa*) among his hirelings, subjects, and throughout his territories.

A play in seven acts

Among the many members of King Life's royal retinue, all of whom are allegorical models for parts of the human mind and body, the principal actors are King Life's wife, Queen Reason (*Buddhi*); the previously mentioned advisors, Worldly Knowledge and Higher Knowledge; and

[20] *Jīvānandanam* Act 3.8–9 (Duraisvāmi Ayyaṅgār 1947: 137–8):
ātmānaṃ parirakṣya duṣkaratapovṛddhadvijārādhanair
dānīyeṣu ca bhaktipūrvam asakṛddeyapradānair api|
daṇḍaṃ daṇḍayitavyamātraviṣayaṃ kṛtvā dharitrītale
rājñā dharmapathe matiṃ kramayatā saṃrakṣitavyāḥ prajāḥ|| 8 ||
kiṃ bahunā
śvaḥśreyasārthaṃ yatate 'niśaṃ yo rājñā kilānena pṛthagvimarṣaḥ|
svasminnamātyeṣu suhṛtsu rāṣṭre durgeṣu kośeṣu baleṣu kāryaḥ|| 9 ||

the *bhakti-guru* Devotion-to-Śiva. King Life's archrival is King Disease, who oversees an allegorical army of disease-soldiers, including Queen Cholera (*Viṣūcī*), Crown Prince Pallid (*Pāṇḍu*), Goiter (*Galagaṇḍa*), Piles (*Arśāṃsi*), Vomiting (*Chardi*), and a host of other insalubrious villains.

Act One opens with a formulaic benediction by the *sūtradhāra*, or stage manager. He offers several laudatory verses to Ānandarāya and a brief description of Ānandarāya's family history, after which the story proper opens in the royal fortress of King Life. The storyline begins with a conversation between Worldly Knowledge and one of his lieutenants, Concentration (*Dhāraṇā*), who, still wearing the disguise of an ascetic, recounts her undercover work inside King Disease's citadel. She tells Worldly Knowledge that King Disease is conspiring with his army to oust King Life from his fortress-body. Concentration's assessment of King Disease's plan and immense might does not bode well for King Life's future welfare.

The play then shifts back and forth between the two kingdoms of Life and Disease. In Act Two, in the kingdom of King Disease, Crown Prince Pallid rallies his troops to discuss their upcoming attack on King Life. King Disease's doorman, Goiter, and some minor lieutenants, Leprosies (*Kuṣṭhāḥ*), Madness (*Unmāda*), Ulcers (*Vraṇāḥ*), Piles (*Arśāṃsi*), and others voice their desire to annihilate King Life and his army. The most vocal of the lot are Diarrhea (*Atīsāra*), whose purported expertise is the unstoppable ability to break through any body's defenses, and Abdominal Tumor (*Gulma*), who boasts that once he gets inside Life's fortress his malignancy will be swift and sure.

In Acts Three and Four, the attack on Life's fortress-body by King Disease's army is well underway. Meanwhile, one of King Disease's spies, Ear Root (*Karṇamūla*), reports that King Life has absconded to an unknown location. In response to King Disease's bombardment, King Life and Queen Reason had retreated to the sanctum sanctorum of King Life's fortress-body, the Lotus City (*Puṇḍarīkapuram*). There they meet Devotion-to-Śiva, who teaches King Life that through devotional surrender to the god Śiva he may obtain a therapeutic brew that will guarantee supreme longevity. This elixir is a medicinal mixture of mercury (*rasa*) and sulphur (*gandhaka*), which is transubstantiated from the semen of Śiva and the menstrual blood of Śiva's consort, Śakti. Under the influence of this brew, no disease can harm the king.

To disrupt King Life's spiritual exercises in the Lotus City, in Act Five, Crown Prince Pallid sends a host of Passions (Envy, Love-and-Hate, Deceit, and Madness) to distract King Life from his meditation. When this fails, Pallid and King Disease fix to target King Life's diet. They send Insalubrity (*Apathyā*) to lure King Life into developing irregular eating habits in the hope that this will make him surrender to two of King Disease's culinary corporals, Overeating (*Atibubhukṣā*) and Bulimia (*Bhasmakā*).

Act Six features a lengthy dialogue between Action (*Karma*) and Time (*Kāla*). They recount the prior events that took place between King Life and his two advisors, Worldly Knowledge and Higher Knowledge. In the course of Action and Time's conversation it is revealed that the efforts of King Disease and Pallid to distance King Life from his two top ministers were partially successful. King Life had apparently become so smitten with Devotion-to-Śiva (a predilection that does not go unnoticed by the king's wife, Reason) that he increased the frequency of their meetings in the Lotus City; during this time he moved away from, nearly to the point of ignoring, the counsel of Worldly

Knowledge, and he relied exclusively on Higher Knowledge for direction. The lopsided attention given to his religious practice has the effect of distracting the king from the material affairs and immediate dangers pressing down on his fortress-body, including the difficulties experienced by all of the people (and bodily components) therein. As far as Higher Knowledge is concerned, this is as it should be. One solely concerned with release from the cycle of rebirth and matters pertaining to ultimate reality need not worry about materiality or threats to the body. Higher Knowledge in this way personifies the philosophical principle of inward-focussed action (*nivṛtti*).

Only when there is nearly complete ruin around him does King Life begin to take stock of what has happened to his fortress-body. After being informed that a legion of diseases has wreaked immense damage on his fortress-body, King Life again accepts the counsel of Worldly Knowledge, who immediately orders and prepares a round of the mercury-sulphur brew earlier handed down from Śiva. He dispenses it to King Life's entire army. This boosts their immuno-defenses against King Disease's attacks, and the healthful troops of King Life ultimately prevail in battle. The action that Worldly Knowledge advises King Life to undertake, contrary to Higher Knowledge's navel-gazing ways, symbolizes the necessity of outwardly focused action, or the principle of *pravṛtti*. On the one hand, he advises King Life to fulfil his body-dharma, symbolized by the ingestion of the Śaiva elixir to enhance bodily immunity; on the other hand, he then urges King Life to accomplish the king's political and martial duties of defending his kingdom.

In Act Seven, with King Disease and his cohort defeated, Worldly Knowledge advises King Life to revisit Devotion-to-Śiva to continue his religious exercises. King Life goes to her, and during his devotional practice, Śiva and Śakti appear before him. Pleased with the king's devotion, the god and goddess grant him pure knowledge of Yoga, the practice of which, they tell him, will enable him to obtain knowledge of the self (*ātman*) and absolute reality (*brahman*). Following the full attainment of this knowledge, the king will be freed from pain, disease, and suffering in this lifetime.

In the end, the actual source of King Life's "disease," that which truly ails him, is the complexity that comes from being human and having to square oneself equally as a body and a self (*śarīra* and *ātman*), that is, as an embodied self. The view of the advisor Worldly Knowledge is that the highest goal of a king's dharma is the establishment of prosperity among the many elements of his *puraṃ* – a Sanskrit word meaning both "fortress" and "body," that Ānandarāya deftly uses throughout the play to refer simultaneously to the king's anatomical body and his royal fortress. King Life cannot create prosperity among the masses until he achieves health in his own body (*puram*), however. Whereas Worldly Knowledge tries to keep King Life grounded and focused on matters of the body-*puram* so that he can then gainfully support the health of the body politic, the religious practices that King Life learns from his other advisor, Higher Knowledge, and his yogic guru, Devotion-to-Śiva (*Śivabhakti*), involve therapies for his individual self (*ātman*), which in turn give his body motivation, focus, and energy to act on behalf of the people of his fortress-*puram*.

Freedom from disease and suffering – well-being – is the "joy of life" of the play's title. Life is joyful, Ānandarāya's play advises, for people who thoroughly understand themselves as embodied entities with important duties (Skt. *dha-*

rmas) to perform in society. Indeed, to adequately execute these socio-religious duties, a person's body must be fit. By virtue of being human, all people are essentially patients in the biophysiological sense, for human bodies are apt to require care at any given point in a lifetime. And while all people are patients because of their embodiment, they are also patients insofar as, once physical health is achieved, people need direction about how to use their bodies in society. But if we are all patients in Ānandarāya's allegorical example, every one of us is also capable of being his or her own physician. After all, there isn't a more consistently available custodian for the body than oneself. Yet, in view of King Life's deliberations about his embodiment and dharmic responsibilities, Ānandarāya makes the case that to be one's own physician, especially in times of acute distress, it is always best to have trustworthy consultants at hand (Worldly Knowledge first and foremost and, secondarily, Devotion-to-Śiva and Higher Knowledge). The lesson to be taken away from this play is that the medicine of Ayurveda is designed to create healthy bodies that permit mental clarity and self-knowledge so that, ultimately, people can be dharmically productive members of society. Health of the physical body, mind, and society jointly constitute the warp and woof of *The Joy of Life*.

References

Bailey, Greg 1985. *Materials for the Study of Ancient Indian Ideologies:* Pravṛtti *and* Nivṛtti, vol. XIX of *Collana di Letture diretta da Oscar Botto*. Torino: Indologica Taurinensia.

Cerulli, Anthony 2007. *Somatic Lessons: Myth and the Body in Sanskrit Medical Literature*. Phd, The University of Chicago.

— forthcoming. "Religio-Medical Perspectives on the

Body, Self and Embodiment in Āyurveda." In B. Holdrege and K. Pechilis (eds.), *Refiguring the Body: Embodiment in South Asian Religions*. Albany: State University of New York Press.

Chattopadhyaya, Debiprasad 1986. "Tradition of Rationalist Medicine in Ancient India: Case for a Critical Analysis of the Caraka-saṃhitā." In Wolfgang Morgenroth (ed.), *Sanskrit and World Culture: Proceedings of the Fourth World Sanskrit Conference of the International Association of Sanskrit Studies, Weimar, May 23–30, 1979*, Schriften zur Geschichte und Kultur des alten Orients, pp. 569–78. Berlin: Akademie-Verlag.

Duraisvāmi Ayyaṅgār, Me. (ed.) 1947. *Jīvānandanam: Āyurvedaśāstratattvaprakaṭanaparaṃ prācīnaṃ nāṭakam. Ānandarāyamakhī praṇītam...Duraisvāmi Ayyaṅgār mahāśayena savimarśaṃ sapariṣkāraṃ ca saṃśodhitam tenaiva viracitayā vipulayā Nandinyākhyayā vyākhyā ca sametam = Jīvānandanam of Ānandarāya Makhin. A Drama Embodying Teachings of Ayurveda, edited by M. Duraiswami Aiyangar...with his own commentary* Nandinī, vol. 59 of *Adyar Library Series*. Madras: Adyar Library.

Dvivedī, Durgāprasāda and Kāśīnātha Pāṇḍuraṅga Paraba (eds.) 1891. *Jīvānandanam Ānandarāyamakhipraṇītaṃ. Paṇḍitadurgāprasādaśarmaṇā, Parabopāhvapāṇḍuraṅgātmajakāśīnāthaśarmaṇā ca saṃśodhitam*, vol. 27 of *Kāvyamālā*. Mumbayyāṃ: Nirṇayasāgarākhyamudraṇālaye, 1st edn. 2nd edition 1933.

Engler, Steven 2003. "'Science' vs. 'Religion' in Classical Ayurveda." *Numen*, **50(4)**, 416–63.

Geertz, Clifford 1973. *The Interpretation of Cultures*. New York: Basic Books.

Kuppuswamy Sastri, T. S. 1904. "Ramabhadra Dikshita and the Southern Poets of his Time." *Indian Antiquary*, **33**, 126–

42, 176–96.

Lupton, Deborah 2003. *Medicine as Culture: Illness, Disease and the Body in Western Societies*. London: Sage, 2nd edn. First edition in 1994.

Meulenbeld, Gerrit Jan 1999–2002. *A History of Indian Medical Literature*, vol. XV of *Groningen Oriental Studies*. Groningen: E. Forsten. 5v.

Nambiar, Sita K. 1998. *Prabodhacandrodaya of Kṛṣṇa Miśra (Sanskrit Text with English Translation, a Critical Introduction and Index)*. Delhi: Motilal Banarsidass, 2nd edn. First edition 1971.

Nārāyaṇadatta, Vaidya (ed.) 1933. *Jīvānandanam Śrīmadānandarāyamakhinpraṇītaṃ...with an introduction by Paṇḍita Śrī Hariśāstrī Dādhīcaḥ*. Khurja, U. P.: Vaidya Nārāyaṇadatta.

Raghavan, V. (ed.) 1952. *Śāhendra Vilāsa, a Poem on the Life of King Śāhaji of Tanjore (1684–1710), of Śrīdhara Veṅkaṭeśa (Ayyāvāl)*, vol. 54 of *Tanjore Sarasvati Mahal Series*. Tiruchi: The Kalyan Press for the TMSSM Library, Tanjore.

Rāmā, Goparājū (ed.) 1991. *Vidyāpariṇayam*. Rashtriya Sanskrit Sansthan, No. 30. Allahabad: Gaṅgānātha Jhā Kendrīya Saṃskṛtavidyāpīṭham.

Sastry, Alladi Mahadeva (ed.) 2001. *Bhagavad Gita, with the Commentary of Adi Sri Sankaracharya*. Chennai: Samata Books, 13th edn. First edition 1918.

Schetelich, Maria 1984. "Niti in Anandarayamakhis Drama "Jivanandana"." *Altorientalische Forschungen*, **11**, 299–330.

Shekhar, I. 1960. *Sanskrit Drama: Its Origin and Decline*, vol. 7 of *Orientalia Rheno-Traiectina*. Leiden: E. J. Brill.

Subramanian, K. R. 1928. *The Maratha Rajas of Tanjore*. Madras: The Author. Reprinted, New Delhi: Asian Educational Services, 1988.

Thapar, Romila 2002. *Early India: From the Origins to AD 1300*. London: Allen Lane. First published 2001.

Vallauri, Mario 1929. *Il Jīvānanda (La felicità dell'anima) di Ānandarāyamakhin*. Lanciano: G. Carabba.

Vyasacharya, Mudgal (ed.) 1881. *Jīvānandanam*. Mysore: Savidyā Mandira Press. Telugu script.

Weckerling, Adolf 1937. *Das Glück des Lebens, medizinisches Drama des Ānandarāyamakhī; zum ersten Male aus dem Sanskrit ins Deutsche übersetzt*. Greifswald: Universitätsverlag Ratsbuchhandlung L. Bamberg.

Zimmer, Heinrich 1979. *Hindu Medicine*. New York: Arno Press. First published in 1948.

Zysk, Kenneth G. 1991. *Asceticism and Healing in Ancient India: Medicine in the Buddhist Monastery*. New York, Bombay, etc.: Oxford University Press. Reprinted, Delhi 1998 and 2000.

6

Kenneth G. Zysk

An Indologist Looks at Siddha Medicine in Tamilnadu

Three traditional medicinal systems predominate in modern India: Ayurveda, Siddha, and Unānī. Ayurveda is found mostly in northern India and in Kerala in the South, Siddha medicine occurs in Tamilnadu and parts of Kerala, and Unānī, which derives from Arabic medicine, is found throughout India, mainly in the urban areas. This essay focuses on Siddha medicine (Tamil *Citta Vaittiyam*) and its history and practice in South India, with an eye towards the similarities and differences between Siddha medicine and Ayurveda.

Research into Siddha medicine in Tamilnadu has revealed certain problems which must be overcome in order to reach a proper understanding of this medical system and its history. The central problem lies with the reliability of the secondary sources, which are written primarily by Tamil Citta doctors. Very little scholarship on the subject has been carried out by western students and scholars of India and Indian medicine.

Due to the increased appreciation of Tamilnadu's uniqueness in South Asia over the past decades, a strong subnationalist movement has grown up in Tamilnadu. Tamilians consider their cultural and linguistic heritage to be older and more important than their Indo-Aryan neighbours to the north; some even claim that their ancestors were the first civilised humans on the planet. The fire of this controversy has recently been kindled by a debate centering on the still-to-be-deciphered script of the so-called Indus Valley Civilisation. This ancient urban culture, whose major cities were located along the banks of the Indus River and its tributaries in what is now Pakistan and parts of Gujarat, resembled the great civilisations of ancient Egypt and Mesopotamia in size, development and age. One side of the debate maintains that the script represents a language probably of Dravidian origin, while the other side claims that it does not represent a language at all. Tamilians, whose language is Dravidian, are anxiously following the debate, for if the former side prevails, it would confirm their antiquity on the Indian subcontinent. In short, the cultural lens through which Tamilians look at their own history can sometimes distort the image in favour of Tamil superiority and antiquity.

History

A few references to Ayurveda are found early in Tamil literature. The Tamil term for Ayurveda, *āyulvetar*, occurs in the *Cilappatikāram*, which is said to date from the mid-fifth century CE; and mention of the three humours (*tiritocam*, Skt. *tridoṣa*) is found in the *Tirukkuṛaḷ*, dating from 450–550 CE.

The first Tamil Siddha text is the *Tirumantiram* by Tirumūlar, whose date is probably the 6th or 7th century CE. In it, there is mention of alchemy used to transform iron into gold; but no specific references to Tamil medicinal doctrines are found. Most critical scholars of Siddha, however, agree that on the basis of their language, the numerous texts on Siddha medicine, which present it as a codified system of healing, cannot be older than the 16th century. We must, therefore, understand that Tamil Siddha, as it is now conceived to be in theory and practice, began in Tamilnadu around the 16th century, but elements of healing practices which eventually became part of Siddha medicine, including those they hold in common with Ayurveda, derive from an earlier period.

Like all systems of Hindu knowledge, Siddha attributes its origin to a divine source; hence its knowledge is sacred and eternal, passed down to humankind for the benefit of all humanity. According to tradition, the god Śiva transmitted the knowledge of medicine to his consort Pārvatī, who in turn passed it on Nandī, from whom it was given successively to the remaining 17 Siddhars, who are the acknowledged traditional transmitters of Siddha medical doctrines and practices. By attributing a divine or extra-human origin to its medicine, the Tamil Siddhars have assured it a legitimate place in the corpus of Hindu knowledge and Tamil literature.

The principles of Siddha medicine

Siddha medicine relies entirely on Ayurveda for the medical doctrines that bridge the natural world and the human body. First, there are the five gross elements (*pañcamahābhūtam*), which make up the entire natural world: solid/earth, fluid/water, radiance/fire, gas/wind, and ether/space. These combine in certain ways to give the three bodily humours (wind, bile, and phlegm), called *muppini* in modern Tamil.

As in Ayurveda, Siddha medicine maintains that the three humours predominate in humans in accordance with their nature and stages of life. Every individual is born with a unique configuration of the three humours, called the person's basic nature, which is fixed at birth and forms the basis of his or her normal, healthy state. However, it is natural that one humour should dominate during the three different stages of life. The classification of the humours in relation to the stages of life in Siddha differs from that found in Ayurveda. According to Siddha, wind predominates in the first third, bile in the second third, and phlegm in the last third of life, while in Ayurveda phlegm dominates the first third and wind the last third of one's life. That is the reason, according to Ayurveda, that as we become older, we tend to develop a tendency to produce more gas in the stomach and bowels.

Diagnosis in Siddha medicine

The diagnosis of disease in Siddha relies on the examination of eight anatomical features (*envagi thaervu*), which are evaluated in terms of the three humours. Of these, most modern Siddha doctors place the greatest emphasis on the examination of the pulse, whereby both diagnosis and prognosis are evaluated at the same time. This method of diagnosis also occurs in Ayurvedic texts, but only after the 14th century. Prior to this time, Ayurvedic treatises teach that diagnosis of disease caused by a disturbance of one or more of the humours is to be carried out by means of observation, touch and interrogation.

Siddha pulse diagnosis (*nāṭīparītchai*, Skt. *nāḍīparīkṣā*), like that found in Ayurveda, in all probability owes its origins to Unānī medicine, where it is a highly developed form of diagnosis derived from Arabic medicine. Moreover, it requires a highly refined sense of touch and subjective awareness, which we call intuition.

The pulse is felt on the female's left and male's right hand by the doctor's opposite hand, a couple of centimetres below the wrist joint using the index, middle, and ring fingers. Pressure should be applied by one finger after the other beginning with the index finger. Each finger represents a particular humour which in normal conditions has a movement representative of certain animals. The index finger feels the windy humour, which should have the movement of a swan, cock, or peacock; the middle finger feels the bilious humour, which should have the movement of a tortoise or a leach; and the ring finger feels the phlegmatic humour, which should have the movement of a frog or a snake. Any deviation from these normal movements indicates which humour or humours are vitiated. If all humours are affected the pulse is usually rapid with a greater volume of blood-flow. After long periods of practice under the guidance of a skilled teach, a student can begin to detect subtle differences in the flow, volume, and speed of the pulse at the point of each of the three finger-tips. These changes correspond to abnormalities in particular body parts, which the skilled Siddha doctor can pinpoint and for which he or she can prescribe the appropriate cure.

The principles of treatment in Siddha medicine

Treatment and pharmaceutics are the two areas where Siddha differs from Ayurveda. Derived from Siddha yoga, the principle aim of Siddha medicine is to make the body a perfectly functioning organism, not subject to the normal process of decay, so that a maximum length of life is achieved. Like Ayurveda, Siddha places emphasis on positive health, so that the primary object of the medicine is disease-prevention. Beyond this fundamental agreement between the two systems, Siddha and Ayurveda differ from each other.

Unlike in Ayurveda, surgery *per se* does not form a significant part of Siddha medicine. Medicated oils and pastes are applied to treat wounds and ulcers, but the use of a knife is not found in Siddha medicine.

Closely connected with the tradition of the martial arts in South India, there developed a treatment by at type of acupressure based on the vital points in the human body, known as *varmam* (Skt. *marman*). There are 107 points mentioned in the Ayurvedic classics, where they are identified and explained as the vulnerable points on the body. Injury to them normally results in death. Although the number can vary, Siddha usually counts 108 out of a total of 400 *varmam* points. Siddha doctors developed techniques of applying pressure to these special points to remove certain aliments and massaging the points to cure diseases. They also specialised in bone-setting and often practised an Indian form of the martial arts, called *cilampam*.

According to Dr Brigitte Sébastia, who has discovered through her fieldwork that the art of *varmam* is particularly widespread among the hereditary Siddha practitioners belonging to the Nādār or Shānār caste in the district of Kanyakumari in southern Tamilnadu. The development of this special form of healing evolved naturally from the males' occupation as toddy-drawers, which necessitated that they climb coconut and palm trees to collect the sap. In carrying out their work, they occasionally fell from great heights. In order to repair the injury or to save the life of a fall-victim, skills of bone-setting and reviving an unconscious patient by massage developed among certain families within the caste, who have passed down their special art from generation to generation by word of mouth. In the past, rulers employed members of this caste to cure injuries incurred in battle and to overpower their enemies by their knowledge of the Indian martial arts.

The Siddha system of rejuvenation-therapy, known as *kāyakalpa* (lit. "making the body competent for long life"), is closely connected to the practice of Siddha yoga and marks the most distinctive feature of Siddha medicine. It involves a five-step process for rejuvenating the body and prolonging life:

1. the preservation of vital energy by means of the yogic technique of breath-control (*vasiyogam* or Skt. *prāṇāyāma*),
2. the conservation of semen,
3. the use of *muppu*,
4. the use of calcinated powders (*chunnam*, Skt. *bhasma*) prepare from metals and minerals, and
5. the use of drugs prepared from plants special to each Siddha doctor.

The esoteric substance called *muppu* is particular to Siddha medicine and may be considered as Siddha's equivalent of the "philosopher's stone" in Western alchemy. Its preparation is hidden in secrecy, known solely by the guru and passed on to the student only when he is ready to receive it. It is generally thought to consist of three salts (*mu-uppu*) called *pūnīru*, *kallupu*, and *vediyuppu*, which correspond respectively to the sun, moon, and fire. *Pūnīru* is called a certain kind of limestone, composed of globules that are found underneath Fuller's Earth. It is collected only on the full-moon night in April, when it is said to bubble out from the limestone, and is then purified with a special herb. *Kallupu* is hard salt or stone salt, i.e., rock salt, which is dug up from mines under the earth, or is obtained from saline deposits under the sea; or else it can be gathered from the froth of sea water, which carries the undersea saline. It is considered to be useful in consolidating mercury and other metals. Finally, *Vediyuppu* is potassium nitrate, which is cleaned seven times and purified with alum.

This religio-medical form of therapy is the cornerstone of the Siddha medical practice and provides the basis for the rich variety of alchemical preparations that make up the pharmacopeia of Siddha medicine.

Alchemy and Siddha pharmacopeia

The precise origin of the system of Siddha pharmacology is not known, but it seems to have been closely linked to the Tantric religious movement, which can be traced back to the 6th century CE in North India and influenced both Buddhism and Hinduism. It was strongly anti-Brahminical and stressed ascetic practices and religious rituals that involved "forbidden" foods and drinks, and sexual intercourse, and often included the use of alchemical preparations.

The alchemical part of Siddha appears from at least the time of Tirumūlar's *Tirumantiram* (6th or 7th century CE), in which various alchemical preparations are mentioned. Alchemy is also found in Sanskrit texts from North India, but from about 6th – 7th centuries CE, and only later became an integral part of Ayurvedic medicine called *Rasaśāstra*, "Traditional knowledge about Mercury." In the classical treatises of Ayurveda, reference to alchemy is wanting and only certain metals and minerals are mentioned in the late classical treatises of the 7th century CE by the author Vāgbhaṭa. Since alchemy plays a more central role in Siddha medicine than it does in Ayurveda, some scholars believed that medical alchemy may well have begun in South India, among the Siddha yogins and ascetics, and was later assimilated into Ayurveda.

Mercury and sulphur are, as in *Rasaśāstra*, the cornerstones of Siddha pharmacology and have been equated to the deities Śiva and Pārvatī. The crucial ingredient in almost every Siddha alchemical preparation is mercury or quicksilver. Although mercury plays a key role in both the Ayurveda and Siddha, it does not occur in its pure form in India and, therefore, must be imported, most often, I am told, from Italy. A prudent student of Siddha medicine is, therefore, compelled to ask: if mercury never existed in its pure form in India, from where did alchemy come?

When combining drugs, Siddha considers substances that form a natural affinity to each other, such as borax and ammonia sulphate, to be greater than the sum of its individual parts, and called it *nādabindu*, where *nāda* is acidic and *bindu* is alkaline, or in the Siddha cosmology female Śakti mated with male Śiva. The most important mixture of this kind is alkaline mercury and acidic sulphur.

The six pharmaceutical preparations are common to both Siddha and Ayurveda, which can be administered internally or topically: calcinated metals and minerals (*chunnam*), powders (*churanam*), decoctions (*kudinir*), pastes (*karkam*), medicate clarified butter (*nei*), and medicate oils (*ennai*).

Both Rasaśāstra and Siddha have devised a method for purifying or detoxifying metals and minerals, called *suddhi murai* in Tamil and *śodhana* in Sanskrit, before they are reduced to ash (*chunnam/bhasma*). However, their techniques and procedures are different. Purification is done by one of two methods in Siddha. One involves the repeated heating of sheets of metal and plunging them into various vegetable juices and decoctions. The other method, called "killing" (*maraṇa*), entails the destroying of the metal or mineral by the use of powerful herbs, so that it loses its identity and becomes converted into fine powders, having the nature of oxides or sulphides, which can by processed by the intestinal juices. After this purification procedure, the metal or mineral is combined with its appropriate acid or alkaline and is then ready for its final transformation into an ash or *bhasman* by incineration in special furnaces made of cowdung cakes.

The incineration process may vary slightly among the different Siddha doctors, but all procedures require repeated heating in a fire fuelled by dung cakes. The number of burnings can reach 100 for certain preparations. In Ayurveda, the duration and intensity of the heat is regulated by the size of the pile of dung cakes called *puṭa*s. Siddha medicine has devised a method with a special substance made of inorganic salts, called *jayanī*, which reduces the number of burnings to only three or four. In order to increase the potency of the *chunnam*, Siddha practitioners add the esoteric substance *muppu*.

Despite the irrefutable scientific evidence that shows most of these minerals and metals to be toxic to the human body, both Ayurvedic and Siddha practitioners continue to use them in their every day practice. They claim that their respective traditions have provided special techniques to detoxify the metals and minerals and to make them extremely potent medicines.

Conclusions

Unlike Ayurveda, which has a long and detailed textual tradition in Sanskrit from around the beginning of the Common Era, Siddha medicine's textual history in Tamil is vague and uncertain until about the 16th century CE, when definitive medical treatises began to appear. Most of the knowledge about Siddha medicine comes from these late Tamil works and from modern-day practitioners, who often maintain a historically unverified development of their own tradition and who, sometimes out of their Tamil enthusiasm, tend to make fantastic claims about the age and importance of Siddha medicine vis-à-vis Ayurveda.

Based on the evidence thus far marshalled by means of written secondary sources and the reports of fieldworkers in Siddha medicine and informed by my own observations, it would appear that Siddha and Ayurveda share a common theoretic foundation, but differ most strikingly in their respective forms of therapeutics. This would tend to suggest that the original form of Siddha medicine consisted principally in a series of treatments for specific aliments, probably derived from regional traditions of folk medicine. Eventually a theoretical framework and epistemology was added to these indigenous forms of medical therapy. The theoretical part of Siddha medicine relies principally on Ayurveda, while its use of pulse (as well as urine) as a means of diagnosing disease owes its origin to the Arabic based Unānī medicine, which was also probably the basis of pulse-diagnosis in Ayurveda.

The core of Siddha medicine is its alchemy, whose fundamental principles conform to those found in the alchemical traditions of ancient Greece and China, and in Arabic alchemy. It would, therefore, seem possible that the alchemy found in both Siddha and Ayurveda could well have derived from one or a combination of these extra-Indian traditions. Further investigation into the principles and practices of each of the ancient systems in relationship to Indian alchemy (both Siddha and Ayurveda) could reveal important connections between Indian and other systems of alchemy and medicine.

Ayurveda has left the soil of India and has found fertile ground in the West, where alternative and complementary forms of healing have become increasingly more popular over the last couple of decades. There are clear signs on the horizon that Siddha medicine is ready to follow the same course. These Indian systems of medicine must undergo changes and adaptations to be accommodated in a foreign environment; and some of these modifications will invariably find their way back to India, where they will be reintroduced into the system. Such has been the pattern of medicine in most parts of the world, so that the final chapter on a particular medical history can never really be written. In fact, an understanding of Siddha's medical history can only be seen in light of its change and adaptations over time.

Further reading

Daniel, E. Valentine (1984). "The Pulse as an Icon in Siddha Medicine." In E. Valentine Daniel and Judy F. Pugh (eds.), *South Asian Systems of Healing*, vol. 18 of *Contributions to Asian Studies*, pp. 115–26. Leiden: Brill.

Ganapathy, T. N. (1993). "The Siddha Conception of the Human Body." In *The Philosophy of the Tamil Siddhas*, chap. 5, pp. 115–40. New Delhi: Indian council of Philosophical Research.

Hausman, Gary J. (1996). *Siddhars, Alchemy, and the Abyss of Tradition: "Traditional" Tamil Medical Knowledge in "Modern" Practice*. Phd, University of Michigan, Ann Arbor.

Kardaswamy, Thiru N. (1979). *History of Siddha Medicine*. Madras: s.n.

Natarajan, N. and M. Govindan (1993). *Thirumandiram: A Classic of Yoga and Tantra by Siddhar Thirumoolar*. Kriya Yoga Pubns. 3v.

Pillai, N. Kandaswamy (1979). *History of Siddha Medicine*. Madras: Government of Tamil Nadu.

Ramaswamy, Sumathi (2004). *The Lost Land of Lemuria: Fabulous Geographies, Catastrophic Histories*. Berkeley: University of California Press.

Scharfe, Hartmut (1999). "The Doctrine of the Three Humors in Traditional Indian Medicine and the Alleged Antiquity of Tamil Siddha Medicine." *Journal of the American Oriental Society*, **119(4)**, 609–29.

Subbarayappa, B. V. (1995/6). "South Indian Siddha Medicine: Some Reflections." *Studies in History of Medicine and Science*, **xiv(1–2)**, 75–89.

— (1997). "Siddha Medicine: an Overview." *The Lancet*, **350**, 1841–44.

Subramanian, S. V. and V. R. Madhavan (eds.) (1983). *The Heritage of the Tamils: Siddha Medicine*. Madras: International Institute of Tamil Studies.

Thayanithy, Maithili (2010). *The Concept of Living Liberation in the Tirumantiram*. Phd, University of Toronto, Toronto. URL `http://hdl.handle.net/1807/24384`.

Venkataraman, R. (1990). *A History of the Tamil Siddha Cult*. Madurai: Ennes.

Weiss, Richard S. (2008). "Divorcing Ayurveda: Siddha Medicine and the Quest for Uniqueness." In Dagmar Wujastyk and Frederick M. Smith (eds.), *Modern and Global Ayurveda: Pluralism and Paradigms*, chap. 4, pp. 77–99. New York: SUNY Press.

— (2009). *Recipes for Immortality: Healing, Religion, and Community in South India*. New York: Oxford University Press.

White, David Gordon (1996). *The Alchemical Body: Siddha Traditions in Medieval India*. Chicago: University of Chicago Press.

Zvelebil, Kamil V. (1973). *The Poets of the Powers*. London: Rider.

— (1983). "The Ideological Basis of the Siddha Search for Immortality." In Beatrix Pfleiderer and Guenther D. Sontheimer (eds.), *Sources of Illness and Healing in South Asian Regional Literature*, vol. 8 (1979) of *South Asian Digest of Regional Writing*, pp. 1–9. Heidelberg: South Asia Institute, Dept. of Tropical Hygiene and Public Health, Dept. of Indology, Heidelberg University.

— (1996). *The Siddha Quest for Immortality*. Oxford: Mandrake of Oxford.

7

Manoj Sankara-narayana

Texts and Physicians in Keralan Ayurveda: the Case of the Rescue Clyster

Introduction

In this chapter, I attempt to show the relevance of textual studies to clinical Ayurvedic practice by looking at the case of the Rescue Clyster (*vaitaraṇavasti*), a commonly-practised enema (*vasti*) formulation in Kerala. I consider how the different enema formulations and current variation in clinical practice among Ayurvedic physicians in Kerala reflect the

I offer my *praṇāmas* to my guru, Padmaśrī Dr K. Rajagopalan, who gave back to the Ayurveda community the highly effective *vaitaraṇavasti*. I dedicate this paper to his lotus feet. I also express my sincere gratitude to Dr P. Ram Manohar and the Arya Vaidya Pharmacy, Coimbatore, for providing me with an opportunity to present this paper. My sincere thanks to Dr P. K. Varrier, Dr P. Madhavankutty Varrier and Dr E. Surendran, Arya Vaidya Sala, Kottakkal, for giving me a chance to present my observations on the practice of the rescue clyster in Keralan Ayurveda; Dr P. T. N. Vasudevan Mooss and Dr Narayanan Nambi, S. N. A. Oushadhasala, Thrissur, for providing an opportunity to present my study at the Unni Mooss Dinam Seminar 2010. This paper would not have assumed its current form without the editorial input of Dr Dominik Wujastyk. I am short of words to express my gratitude to him. Last but not least, I wish to express my gratitude to all the members of the Classical Ayurveda Text Study Group (CATS) for motivating us to take up textual studies through their inspiring work.

ways in which Ayurvedic practice arose from established theoretical foundations. I deal with Ayurvedic clinical practice here from both a text-historical perspective and from the perspective of a practicing, clinical physician.

In the following pages, I trace the appearance of the Rescue Clyster (*vaitaraṇavasti*) in the medical literature of Ayurveda up to the present, as well as the current practice of enema among physicians in Kerala. I also consider the extent to which the evolution of contemporary practice is reflected in Ayurvedic literature.[1]

The Rescue Clyster became popular following the research of P. Sankarankutty, M. R. Vasudevan Namboodiri and V. K. Sasikumar at the Government Ayurveda College in 1991.[2] Their work was inspired by Dr K. Rajagopalan's compilation of enema therapies (*vastiyoga*).[3] The practice of this type of enema (*vasti*) varies considerably from institution to institution and from individual to individual. For example, the formulation used for performing the Rescue Clyster in the Government Ayurveda College, Thiruvanantapuram, is in Table 7.1. In the Central Institute of Pañcakarma, Cheruthuruty, 450 ml of *kṣīra* or cow's urine (*gomūtra*) is used, while the measurements for the rest are the same. To make sense of the variations of this practice, a thorough scrutiny of textual references related to its formula is necessary.

The *Carakasaṃhitā* is an important Sanskrit medical source for Ayurvedic clinical practice. According to Caraka,

---

[1] Although care is taken to present the facts objectively, the absence of a systematic codification of clinical research means that the paper may carry some minor misrepresentations regarding the practice of the Rescue Clyster.

[2] Sasikumar *et al.* 1991.

[3] Personal communication with Dr P. Sankarankutty, Dr V. K. Sasikumar, and Dr T. K. Sudarshanan Nair.

sea salt (*saindhava*)	15 g
jaggery (*guḍa*)	30 g
tamarind (*amlikā*)	60 g
sesame oil (*taila*)	120 ml
cow's urine (*gomūtra*)	
or	
thickened milk (*kṣīra*)	240 ml

Table 7.1: *Vaitaraṇavasti* in Thiruvanantapuram

medical practice is far more than mere acquaintance with the healing properties of medicinal herbs.

> Practice depends on time and measure, and success is founded on practice. A person who knows practice always stands at the head of those who know about drugs.[4]

It is elimination therapy (*śodhanacikitsā*), and such therapies that form the basis of Ayurveda. Another work, the *Narasiṃhabhāṣya*, a unique commentary by Narasiṃha on the *Rasavaiśeṣikasūtra*, datable perhaps to the seventh or eighth century CE, has left a great impact on the Ayurveda fraternity of Kerala.[5] In general, this commentary serves as an authoritative interpretation (*vārttika*) applicable to the whole Ayurveda of eight components (*aṣṭāṅgāyurveda*), and specifically to the branch of Ayurveda dealing with internal medicine (*kāyacikitsā*). The *Narasiṃhabhāṣya* reveals the special status enjoyed by internal medicine due to the inclusion of elimination therapies (*pañcakarma*) in this branch.

---

[4]*Carakasaṃhitā Sū* 2.16 (Ācārya 1941: 25b): *mātrākālāśrayā yuktiḥ siddhir yuktau pratiṣṭhitā | tiṣṭhaty upari yuktijño dravyajñānavatāṃ sadā ||* (tr. DW).

[5]On the date of *Narasiṃhabhāṣya*, see Meulenbeld 1999–2002: IIA, 138.

Purificatory therapy (*śodhanacikitsā*), also known as the five-fold elimination therapy (*pañcakarma*), was regarded in high esteem by Narasiṃha, and all branches of Ayurveda utilised the purificatory therapy.[6] In his exhaustive work *A History of Indian Medical Literature* (henceforth *HIML*), Meulenbeld cites only two self-contained, original texts in this regard, both on five-fold elimination therapy (*pañcakarma*), the *Pañcakarmavicāra* and *Pañcakarmavidhi*.[7] Furthermore, manuscript copies of a work entitled *Pañcakarmādhikāra* are found in libraries in Calcutta.[8] The dearth of knowledge among physicians about the ideal practice of *pañcakarma* has created a new scenario in which the procedure of enema itself has created many iatrogenic complications (diseases caused by five-fold elimination therapy).[9]

As a part of the elimination procedure of *pañcakarma*, enema (*vasti*) has been given special status from the classical period onwards. In his *Āyurvedasaukhyaṃ*, Ṭoḍaramalla (*fl. ca.* 1550–1589) refers to a school of thought propounded

[6]See, for example, *Narasiṃhabhāṣya* 1.1 (Muthuswami 1976: 2), asserting the primacy of internal medicine (*kāyacikitsā*) and purificatory regimes: *pūrvaprakṛtā hy atra gṛhītatantraśarīrā viśeṣārthajijñāsavo martyāḥ| teṣām anumatyartham uktam iti| evaṃ vārttikaprayojanam api dyotitaṃ bhavati viśeṣārthaprakāśanam iti| bhavati cātra sūtrārthānām upapattisūcanāt tatparihāravacanaṃ, viśeṣārthadarśanaṃ ca vārttikam iti| atrāha – kasyedaṃ vārttikam iti| aṣṭāṅgasyāyurvedasya sakalasya, ārogyaśāstraṃ vyākhyāsyāma ity aviśeṣeṇoktatvāt sarvatantrapadārthasaṃgrahāc ca| athavā viśeṣataḥ kāyacikitsāyāḥ|*

[7]*HIML*: IIA, 525; cf. Raghavan *et al.* 1949–: 11, 8a. A manuscript of the *Pañcakarmavicāra* in Telugu script is OLM Accession Number P8734/6, Government Oriental Library, Mysore.

[8]Rama Rao (2005: p. 170, serial no. #1741) records four manuscripts: Asiatic Society Calcutta, acc. no. IE 45; Calcutta Sanskrit College Library acc. no. 248, and also acc. nos. 171 and 189 ascribed to a Vijayarakṣita.

[9]*Śārṅgadharasaṃhitā* prathamakhaṇḍa 7, v. 193cd-194ab (Śāstrī 1931: 132): *hīnamithyātiyogena bhedaiḥ pañcadaśoditāḥ| pañcakarmabhavā rogā rogeṣv eva prakīrtitāḥ|*

by Atri that deems enema therapy (*vasticikitsā*) to be an independent, ninth branch of Ayurveda.[10] He explains that enema therapy (*vasticikitsā*) is included under the internal therapy (*kāyacikitsā*) branch of Ayurveda found in the compendia of Caraka and Suśruta.[11] From a textual-historical perspective, this strongly suggests that the practice of enema in Ayurvedic clinical practice is significant.

Vasti in Kerala

The legacy handed down by Kerala's Ayurvedic physicians is a vibrant clinical practice, well-rooted in the fundamental principles of the Sanskrit medical classics. This observation can be established by a cursory examination of Kerala's rich literary tradition, which focuses on the fundamental principles of the Sanskrit medical sources as well as the clinical application of those sources. The literary contribution from Kerala includes various commentaries (especially on the *Aṣṭāṅgahṛdaya Saṃhitā*), treatises on poison treatment (*viṣacikitsā*), paediatrics (*bālacikitsā*), and various other books on clinical practice written in both Sanskrit and mixed Sanskrit and Malayālam (*maṇipravālaṃ*). Yet, the teaching of Ayurveda in Kerala does not contribute much to the schemata of purification therapy (*śodhanacikitsā*).[12] This reminds us of

[10] *Āyurvedasaukhyaṃ* 1.37 (Dash and Kashyap 1992: 61): *atri mate navaprakārikā cikitsā carakasuśrutādibhir viṣopaśamanārthaṃ yā agadā nāma kriyā proktā saivātriṇā basticikitsā kṛtā*|, and 1.38: *gudāmayānāṃ yā bastiḥ śamanaṃ ca nirūhaṃ*| *āsthāpanānuvasaś ca agadaṃ nāma kathyate*|

[11] *Āyurvedasaukhyaṃ* 1.39 (Dash and Kashyap 1992: 62): *suśrutādīnāṃ mate basticikitsā kāyacikitsāntarbhūtaiva*| *ato 'tra mayā na aṃṅgīkāraḥ kṛtaḥ* 39|

[12] For example, in the *Yogāmṛta* (15th–17th century CE, edited by Nambiyār Vaidyar (1960)), a handbook for clinical practice, enema (*vasti*) is used as a therapeutic tool in only six instances: (1) ileus (*udāvarta*), where constipation is experienced even after doing oil massage (*abhyaṅga*), applying a hot poultice (*piṇḍasveda*) and an anal wick (*gudavarti*), enema

the statement by Cakrapāṇidatta (*fl. ca.* 1075), which points to the declining importance of enema in Ayurvedic practice during his period:[13]

> Many formulae for the preparation of enemas that are available in the compendia of Caraka and others were not included in this treatise as they are no longer utilised in current routine clinical practice.

Many formulae for the preparation of enemas that are available in the compendia of Caraka and other preceptors were not elaborated in this treatise as they were no longer utilised in the routine clinical practice by that time. Niścalakara (*fl. ca.* 1150–1200) and Śivadāsasena (*fl. ca.* 1475–1500), commentators on Cakrapāṇidatta's work, explain the word "chiefly" (*prāyo*) as suggestive of the clinical utilisation, in appropriate conditions, from the list of enema compounds (*vastiyoga*) enumerated in the classical treatises. This statement by the commentators does not negate the importance of Cakrapāṇi's observance regarding enema. This bold admission by Cakrapāṇidatta does not mean that later treatises do not add any novel formulae on enema (*vasti*). For example, the *Vṛndamādhava* (also known as *Siddhayoga*, composed ca. 800–950), that preceded Cakrapāṇidatta,

---

has to be carried out (ch. 17, v. 40). (2) When hernial enlargement (*antravṛddhi*) approaches the groin, it is incurable, but can be maintained in a palliable (*yāpya*) state by treatments which also include enema (*vasti*) (29, v. 16). (3) A swelling in the seat of digested food (*pakvāśayagatagulma*) is treated by vasti (30, vv. 1, 6). (4) The application of an enema (*vastikarma*) is indicated in *pakṣāghāta* and *ākṣepaka* (40, vv. 18, 21). (5) In wind attack in the sides and back (*kaṭipṛṣṭagatavāta*), dominated by pain, enema is indicated (40, vv. 46, 48, 49). (6) The application of an enema (*vastikarma*) is also indicated in gripes (*śūla*) (43, v. 17).

[13]*Cikitsāsaṅgraha* 71.34 (Sharma 1993: 864): *carakād yo samuddiṣṭāḥ bastayo ye sahasraśaḥ| vyavahāro na taiḥ prāyo nibaddhā nātra tena te.*

had introduced newer enema formulations of alkali enema (*kṣāravasti*), the Rescue Clyster, etc.

In the recent history of Kerala's Ayurvedic practice, especially in the former princely state of Travancore, laudable contributions have been made in the area of drug studies, clinical researches, and publications by physicians of Certhala Taluk.[14] Their field of interest also included purification therapy (*śodhanacikitsā*), and these physicians published many pioneering works in the field of elimination therapies (*pañcakarma*), such as Pāṇāvalli C. Kṛṣṇanvaidyan's *Vastipradīpam* and Manakoḍaṃ Keśavanvaidyan's *Pañcakarma athavā śodhanacikitsā*.[15] The presence of an uninterrupted Aṣṭavaidya lineage in Kerala that preserved and enhanced Vāgbhaṭa's clinical treatises and the works of the Certhala Taluk physicians gave a new lease on life to the speciality of purification therapy (*śodhanacikitsā*).

P. S. Varier was perhaps the first to write about Ayurvedic therapies specific to Kerala, when he discussed the topic of flow therapy (*dhārā*) in the Malayalam journal *Dhanwantari* in 1906. But the publication of formal literature devoted to the specialised treatment therapeutic procedures of Kerala in all likelihood began in 1913 with the publication of the *Dhārākalpa*.[16] This was followed by P. Raman Menon's *Śrī Śirasekādividhi*,[17] N. S. Mooss's monograph on the specialised treatment procedures of Kerala,[18] and Aryavaidyan S. Raghunatha Iyer's Sanskrit

[14]Eṭṭi Acyutan, a physician hailing from Certhala Taluk, contributed significantly to the compilation of historic work *Hortus Malabaricus* of van Rheede (1678–1703).

[15]Kṛṣṇanvaidyan 1988 and Keśavanvaidyan 1993.

[16]Nīlakaṇṭhaśarma and Ācārya 1913.

[17]Menon 1929/1930.

[18]Mooss 1983.

work on specialised therapies.[19] All of these activities rekindled interest in specialised treatment procedures, including purification therapy (*śodhanacikitsā*), in Ayurvedic practice both within and outside of the state of Kerala.

The Rescue Clyster (*vaitaraṇavasti*), an enema formulation popular among the current generation of Ayurveda clinicians in Kerala, is not mentioned in the abovementioned works related to enema (*vasti*).[20]

Vasti formulations in Vaṅgasena's *Cikitsāsārasaṃgraha*

The enema formulation in the *Cikitsāsārasaṃgraha* by Vaṅgasena (*fl.* 1050–1100) was subjected to study in the abovementioned research.[21] The formula for enema in this text reads:[22]

rock salt (*sindhujanma*)		
or sea salt (*saindhavalavaṇa*)	one *karṣa*	12 g
jaggery (*guḍa*)	half a *pala*	24 g
tamarind (*amlikā*)	one *pala*	48 g
sesame oil (*taila*)	*iṣat taila*	a little
cow's milk (*surabhipayaḥ*)	one *kuḍava*	240 ml

[19] Raghunatha Iyer 1972.

[20] Neither Kṛṣṇanvaidyan (1988) nor Keśavanvaidyan (1993) mention this enema (*vasti*) formulation. Caustic enema (*kṣāravasti*) and the Rescue Clyster were not common in the routine clinical practice of Kerala's Aṣṭavaidya tradition.

[21] For example, by Sasikumar *et al.* 1991.

[22] *Vaṅgasena* bastiprakaraṇa 186–190 (Rāya 1983: 805, Bhaṭṭācārya 1893: 947–48): *sindhūdbhavasya karṣam amlikāyāḥ palaṃ guḍārddhapalaṃ| surabhīpayasaḥ kuḍavaḥ sarvair etaiḥ kṛto bastiḥ||186|| īṣattailayuto 'yaṃ bhukte datte nihanti rogagaṇam| kaṭyūrupṛṣṭhaśothaṃ śūlaṃ cāmānilaṃ ghoram||187|| cirabhavam ūrustambhaṃ gṛdhrasirogaṃ ca jānusaṃkocaṃ| viṣamajvarāṇi ghoraṃ klaibyañ ca vināśayaty āśu||188|| bastir vaitaraṇokto guṇagaṇayuktaḥ suvikhyātaḥ||189|| bhojayitvā ca sāyāhne sarvasyāyaṃ praśasyate| atha ced balavān jantur abhuktvāpi tadā kvacit||190||*

While the present study lacks an exhaustive survey of the textual data to support this formulation, it is clear that the formula was furthermore modified by increasing the quantity of milk to two *kuḍava*. Vaṅgasena's text explains that this increase in the quantity of milk was done to reduce the consistency of the enema so that it can be administered more easily. Sasikumar *et al.* (1991: 105) noted that,

> ...the modalities of mixing the ingredients are not mentioned. The main impediment of combination of tamarind and milk together. Milk will readily coagulate when combined with tamarind. Also honey and kalka are not mentioned. A viable alternate method is adopted by mixing jaggery in water and evaporating required quantity of water so as to make the solution dense to be used as honey. Sea salt is an ingredient and *tila taila* can be used as *sneha*. Tamarind is mixed and squeezed well in hot water to be used as *kalkka*. Milk is boiled well and cooled and added at the end to substitute *kwatha*. The disorganisation is seen very much less when this methodology is followed. The vasti constituted thus will be very thick thus rendering it difficult to negotiate through vasti yantra since only one kuḍava (app. 250 ml) of milk is added.the problem can be settled by adding 2 kuḍavas of milk. The constituted vasti is taken in vasti putaka administered. Vaitarana vasti can be given after food in the afternoon like an anuvasana. But if the patient has adequate strength, it can be administered like a niruha also.

The oil used was 120 ml, or approximately two *palas*.

Confusion regarding the combination of substances in the Rescue Clyster is further complicated when one refers to Śāligrāma Vaiśya's early nineteenth-century Hindi translation of Vaṅgasena's work, that includes cow's urine (*gomūtra*) instead of milk as a necessary constituent.[23] This addition may have been influenced by former medical treatises like *Vṛndamādhava* and *Cakradatta*.[24] This ambiguity created two sections among physicians; the division was based on each physician's choice for one of the liquid ingredients, that is, those who preferred cow's urine (*gomūtra*), and the others who preferred milk (*kṣīra*).

The first textual reference to the Rescue Clyster (*vaitaraṇavasti*) is found in the *Vṛndamādhava* (also called the *Siddhayoga*):[25]

> *kṣāraṃ na ced vaitaranaṃ pradāya dvyahe tryahe vāpy anuvāsanīyaḥ|*

The placement of this enema in the *Vṛndamādhava* is noteworthy. In the Ānandāśrama edition of this text (Pādhye 1894), the Rescue Clyster is explained in an independent section after the section on non-oily enemas (*nirūha*),[26] since this formulation does not satisfy the combination pattern of ingredients observed in the preparation of non-oily en-

[23]Jaina 1996: 1000 (reprint of Jaina 1904).

[24]Jaina 1996: 1000. Cakradatta is placed before Vaṅgasena by some historians.

[25]*Vṛndamādhava* ch. 75.3 (Pādhye 1894: 559; cf. also Tivārī 2007). Commenting on this, Śrīkaṇṭhadatta explains (Pādhye 1894: 559): *yasya virecanaṃ nocitaṃ saṃcitaṃ ca malam asti tasya tanmalāpagamārthaṃ kṣāraṃ vaitaraṇaṃ vā bastiṃ dattvānuvāsanaṃ deyaṃ viśuddhasya snehabastyupadeśāt.*

[26]By contrast, the critical edition of the text by Dr Premvati Tiwari explains it in the non-oily enemas (*nirūha*) section, verses 43–4 (Tivārī 2007).

emas (*nirūhavasti*) (i.e., *mākṣikaṃ, lavaṇaṃ, snehaṃ, kalkaṃ,* and *kvāthaṃ*[27]) and is of lesser quantity.

The formula given by Vṛnda has:[28]

sea salt (*saindhava*)	*karṣa*	12 g
jaggery (*guḍa*)	*śukti*	24 g
tamarind (*amlīkā*)	*pala*	48 g
cow's urine (*gomūtra*)	*kuḍava*	240 ml

The indications of enema formulation are gripes (*śūla*), loose bowels (*anāha*), and windy constipation (*āmavāta*). The critical edition of the *Vṛndamādhava* by Tivārī (2007) reports a variant reading, where jaggery (*guḍa*) is replaced by asafoetida (*hiṅgu*).[29] Ṭoḍaramalla's *Āyurvedasaukhyaṃ* describes the formula of the Rescue Clyster using verses similar to those in Vṛnda's *Vṛndamādhava*.[30] Cakrapāṇidatta also accepts the same formula as Vṛnda.[31] The text of the *Cikitsāsaṅgraha* as printed in the Sharma (1993) edition, accompanying *Niścalakara*'s commentary, omits the term *īṣat*, and reads: *tailayuto 'yaṃ*.[32] But *Niścalakara* seems to

[27] *Aṣṭāṅgahṛdayasaṃhitā* sūtra, 19.45cd–46ab (Kuṃṭe *et al.* 1995: 279): *mākṣikaṃ lavaṇaṃ snehaṃ kalkaṃ kvātham iti kramāt| āvapeta nirūhāṇām eṣa saṃyojane vidhiḥ|*

[28] *Vṛndamādhava* 74.43–4 (or 76.1–2 of the vaitaraṇabasti section in the edition of Pādhye (1894: 576)): *palaśuktikarṣakuḍavair amlīkāguḍasindhujanmagomūtraiḥ| īṣattailayuto 'yaṃ bastiḥ sūlān āhāmavātaharaḥ|| bhojayitvā tu sāyāhne sarvasyāyaṃ praśasyate| atha ced balavāñjantur abhuktvāpi tadā kvacit||*

[29] *Ibid.*, Tivārī 2007: 2, 938: *...amlīkāhiṅgusindhujanmagomūtraiḥ|*

[30] Dash and Kashyap 1980–1992: v. 3, ch. 14, vv. 62–3.

[31] *Cikitsāsaṅgraha* 71.30–31 (Sharma 1993: 863) $\simeq$ (Bhaṭṭācārya and Bhaṭṭācārya 1993: 890–91): *palaśuktikarṣakuḍavair amlīkāguḍasindhujanmagomūtreḥ īṣattailayuto 'yaṃ bastiḥ śūlānāhām avātaharaḥ| vaitaraṇaḥ kṣārabastir bhuktecāpi pradīyate|*

[32] *Cikitsāsaṅgraha* 71.31 (Sharma 1993: 863).

accept the reading *iṣattailayuto 'yaṃ*, as he comments on the term *īṣat*.[33] While commenting on this section, *Niścalakara* offers yet another formula for the Rescue Clyster, that he ascribes to an *Āyurvedasāra*.[34] The formula amounts to the following:

sea salt (*saindhava*)	*akṣa*	12 g
jaggery (*guḍa*)	*pala*	48 g
tamarind (*ciñcā*)	*pala*	48 g
sesame oil (*taila*)	*pala*	48 g
cow's urine (*gomūtra*)	*kuḍava*	240 ml

Commentators on the Sanskrit medical sources offer important clues about the composition of the Rescue Clyster formulations. Śrīkaṇṭhadatta (*fl.* 12th century) and Śivadāsasena (*fl. ca.* 1475), commentators on the *Vṛndamādhava* and *Cikitsāsaṅgraha* respectively, explain that even though a measurement of ingredients for enema should be taken as explained in the textual formulae, nevertheless the quantity of cow's urine (*gomūtra*) should be doubled, in accordance with the general rule of interpretation (*paribhāṣā*) about the doubling of liquid ingredients (*dravadvaigu-*

[33] *Ratnaprabhā* (Sharma 1993: 863): *īṣattailam iti palam iti vyavaharanti vṛddhāḥ|* [Since the omission of '*īṣat*' renders the śloka unmetrical, and the word is present in other editions, this may be a slip in the 1993 edition – ed.]

[34] Niścalakara's *Ratnaprabhāṭīkā* on *Cikitsāsaṅgraha* 71.30-31 (Sharma 1993: 863): *yad uktam āyurvedasāre – gomūtrakuḍavaś caikaś ciñcāguḍapalaṃ palaṃ| satailaṃ saindhavasyākṣam ete vaitaraṇāhvayaḥ| kṛte bhukte prayukto 'yaṃ śothaṃ mandāgnitāṃ jayet| gṛdhrasījānusaṅkocasaṃstambhaṃ viṣamajvaraṃ|* [Sharma (1993: 15) identifies the author of the *Āyurvedasāra*, that Niścala also cites elsewhere, as Acyuta, on whom see Raghavan *et al.* (1949–: 2.153b) – ed.]

ṇyaṃ).[35] In other words, they maintain a tradition of adding double the quantity of liquid ingredients explained in the formulae. Candraṭa explains that this practice of doubling of the quantity of liquid ingredients is appropriate for liquid (*drava*) that has the quantity of *kuḍava* or more.[36] The commentators Niścalakara and Śivadāsasena on Cakrapāṇidatta's *Cikitsāsaṅgraha* stipulate that the quantity of sesame oil (*taila*) is one *pala* (*ca.* 48 g) on the basis of existing tradition (*vṛddhavaidyasammatāt*).[37] Śivadāsasena's *Tattvacandrikāṭīkā* presents the practice of adding one emetic nut (*madanaphala*) to the Rescue Clyster (*vaitaraṇavasti*).[38] This is normally added to every non-oily enema (*nirūhavasti*).[39] This tradition seems to be a conscious effort to grant the status of non-oily enema (*nirūhavasti*) to the Rescue Clyster.

Before further elaborating the enema formulation of Vaṅgasena, it is helpful to look at the term *vaitaraṇa* in the Ayurvedic classics. The term *vaitaraṇa* is used as the proper name of a preceptor of surgery (*śalyatantrācārya*)

---

[35]Śrīkaṇṭhadatta's *Vyākhyākusumāvalī* (Pādhye 1894: 576): *gomūtrasya kuḍavo 'ṣṭau palāni dravadvaiguṇyāt| nirūheṣu rasādīnāṃ pramāṇaṃ tu yathāśrutīti paribhāṣāṃ punar dravadvaiguṇyaniṣedhikāṃ nādriyante|*

[36]Candraṭa on *Cikitsākalikā* v. 82 (Sharma 1987: 54): *mūtrakuḍavadvitayaṃ gomūtrasyāṣṭaupalāni| dviguṇaparibhāṣātra kuḍavād ūrdhvaṃ kriyata iti|*; *Aṣṭāṅgahṛdayasaṃhitā, Kalpasiddhisthāna* 6.23 (Kuṃṭe *et al.* 1995: 775): *dviguṇaṃ yojayed ārdraṃ kuḍavādi tathā dravam|*

[37]*Ratnaprabhāṭīkā* on *Cikitsāsaṅgraha* 71, vv. 30–31 (Sharma 1993: 863): *īṣat tailam iti palam iti vyavaharanti vṛddhāḥ|*; *Tattvacandrikāṭīkā, ibid.* (Bhaṭṭācārya and Bhaṭṭācārya 1993: 891): *īṣat śabdena tailapalam iti vyavaharanti vṛddhāḥ|*

[38]*Tattvacandrikāṭīkā* (Bhaṭṭācārya and Bhaṭṭācārya 1993: 891): *atrāpi madanaphalam ekaṃ deyam ity āhuḥ|*

[39]Candraṭa citing Kharanāda (Sharma 1987: 54): *tathā ca kharanādaḥ – ata ūrdhvaṃ pravakṣyāmi nirūhasya prakalpanam| dvādaśaprasṛtān ādye tato 'nyāṃs tu prakalpayet| sarveṣv eva nirūheṣu madanaṃ ca prakalpayet| snehaṃ guḍaṃ mākṣikaṃ ca lavaṇaṃ cāpi yuktitaḥ|*

in the *Suśrutasaṃhitā*.[40] Some have argued that the name in Vaṅgasena refers to this preceptor Vaitaraṇa. Yet, few references to the works of Vaitaraṇa are seen in the commentaries of Śrīdāsapaṇḍita,[41] or Cakrapāṇidatta.[42] The extrapolation of Preceptor Vaitaraṇa to the context of clinical enema does not help much to round out our understanding of the composition and practice of enema (*vasti*). Instead, I suggest that the term *vaitaraṇa* was coined by Vṛnda as a conventional technical term (*pāribhāṣikasaṃjñā*).[43] Vaṅgasena seems to be making an obvious reference to the Rescue Clyster (*vaitaraṇavasti*) mentioned in previous treatises like the *Vṛndamādhava*, when he uses the phrase "together with the collection of qualities mentioned for a *vaitaraṇa*" (*vaitaraṇoktaguṇagaṇayuktaṃ*).[44] And his adjective "famous" (*suvikhyāta*) at the same place appears to be an acknowledgement of its time-tested usage and acceptance among physicians.

Vaṅgasena contends that his substitution of cow's urine (*gomūtra*) (which has the pungent taste (*kaṭurasa*) and the

[40] *Suśrutasaṃhitā, sūtrasthāna* 1, 3 (Ācārya 1938: 1).

[41] Śrīdāsapaṇḍita (14th century) commenting on the *Aṣṭāṅgahṛdayasaṃhitā, sūtrasthāna*, 1.14 (Mooss 1940: 47): *vaitaraṇenāpy uktam – 'prāṇināṃ mūlam āhāraḥ śarīropacayasya sa … raseṣu sadāyatto rasā dravyāśritāḥ smṛtāḥ'*| and he also quotes a *Vetaraṇa* in *sūtra* 20.16: *uktaṃ ca vetaraṇena – raktapittavikāreṣu pittaprakṛtaye tathā| kāle coṣṇe viśeṣeṇa vinā svedaṃ prayojayet|*

[42] See Cakrapāṇidatta's comments on *Suśrutasaṃhitā* sū.18.9–11 and 17–18 (Ācārya and Śarman 1939: 139, 141). [On Vaitaraṇa as a person, see further Meulenbeld 1999–2002: IA, 371 – ed.]

[43] A *pāribhāṣikasaṃjñā* is a technical term that directly refers to an object and has neither a generic feature (*jāti*) nor an attribute (*upādhi*) as the basis of reference.

[44] See note 22 above, v. 189. A syntactic analysis (*vigraha*) of the term *vaitaraṇokta* would be *vaitaraṇāya uktaṃ* in the dative case (*caturthīvibhakti*), and not "stated by Vaitaraṇa" (*vaitareṇe uktaṃ*) using the instrumental (*tṛtiyā*).

dry, non-oily quality (*rūkṣaguṇa*)) with cow's milk (*gokṣīrā*) – which is sweet (*madhura*) and viscous (*snigdha*) – will not alter the clinical efficacy of the popular Rescue Clyster (*vaitaraṇavasti*). This modification seems to be done to suit the patient, who is in a state where oil depletion (*rūkṣatā*) predominates and strength (*bala*) is reduced. Candraṭa advises that when physicians perform an oil-depletion enema (*rūkṣavasti*) in cases associated with obstruction (*āvaraṇa*) and in unobstructed (*nirāvaraṇa*) conditions, the enema (*vasti*) should be prepared by adding one *pala* (48 g) of sesame oil (*taila*).[45] Āḍhamalla, the commentator on the *Śārṅgadharasaṃhitā*, who closely follows Vaṅgasena, refers to the enema (*vasti*) preparation as Milk Rescue Clyster (*kṣīravaitaraṇaṃ*).[46] This substantiates my hypothesis that Vaṅgasena modified the Rescue Clyster (*vaitaraṇavasti*) by substituting cow's urine (*gomūtra*) with cow's milk (*gokṣīrā*).

Formulæ for *vaitaraṇavasti* available from various treatises and commentaries

Formula 1

According to the reading of *Vṛndamādhava*, the *Cikitsāsaṅgraha*, and the *Āyurvedasaukhya*, the ingredients are:

---

[45]Candraṭa, commenting on *Cikitsākalikā* 82 (Sharma 1987: 54): *sāvaraṇe rūkṣam| nirāvaraṇe tailapalānvitaṃ|*

[46]Āḍhamalla, commenting on *Śārṅgadharasaṃhitā* uttarakhaṇḍa 5.16-18 (Śāstrī 1931: 323): *yasya ca virecanaṃ nocitaṃ saṃcitaṃ ca malaṃ bastiṃ tasya ca tanmalāpagamārthakṣiravaitaraṇaṃ vā bastiṃ dattvānuvāsanaṃ deyaṃ| triśuddhasya snehavastyupadeśāt|* It is interesting to note that Āḍhamalla closely follows Śrīkaṇṭhadatta, but replaces the term *vaitaraṇa* ("clyster") with *kṣīravaitaraṇa* ("milk-clyster").

sea salt (*saindhava*)	*karṣa*	12 g
jaggery (*guḍa*)	*śukti*	24 g
tamarind (*amlikā*)	*pala*	48 g
sesame oil (*taila*)	*īṣat*	small amount
cow's urine (*gomūtra*)	*kuḍava*	240 ml

FORMULA 2

According to the variant reading of the *Vṛndamādhava*, jaggery (*guḍa*) is replaced by *hiṅgu*:

sea salt (*saindhava*)	*karṣa*	12 g
hiṅgu	*śukti*	24 g
tamarind (*amlikā*)	*pala*	48 g
sesame oil (*taila*)	*īṣat*	small amount
cow's urine (*gomūtra*)	*kuḍava*	240 ml

FORMULA 3

According to the *Āyurvedasāra* of Acyuta:

sea salt (*saindhava*)	*karṣa*	12 g
jaggery (*guḍa*)	***pala***	48 g
tamarind (*amlikā*)[47]	*pala*	48 g
sesame oil (*taila*)	***pala***	48 g
cow's urine (*gomūtra*)	*kuḍava*	240 ml

[47]Śivadāsasena, commenting on caustic enema (*kṣāravasti*), explains the term *amlikā* as the *amlikāyā iti sāstitintiḍiphalasya* that is to take the tamarind (*amlikā*) along with its seeds. This is not seen in practice in Kerala.

We can stipulate the quantity of sesame oil (*taila*) is one *pala* on the basis of the *Niścalakara* and the *Śivadāsa*. Regarding the quantity of cow's urine (*gomūtra*), *Niścalakara* is silent; but both *Śrīkaṇṭhadatta* and *Śivadāsa* take it as eight *palas* (*aṣṭapala-*) by sticking to the rule of interpretation (*paribhāṣā*) concerning double-measures of fluids (*dravadvaiguṇya*).

1. Formula 1 is further modified by adding one emetic nut (*madanaphala*) to the enema formulation in line with the tradition quoted by *Śivadāsa*.
2. In the compendium of Vaṅgasena, where the cow's urine (*gomūtra*) is replaced by *gokṣīra*.

In our clinical experience we observed that the use of one *pala* of sesame oil (*taila*), rather than the current practice of taking two *palas* of sesame oil (*taila*), has resulted in better outcomes.[48] This demands a well-designed study of various formulations of *vaitaraṇavasti* for establishing its relative clinical efficacy and thereby standardising the formula of *vaitaraṇavasti*.

Indication

The number of conditions where Rescue Clyster (*vaitaraṇavasti*) is therapeutically indicated increases in texts that come after Vaṅgasena, as shown in Table 7.3. And we can see a similar increase in conditions indicated for treatment

[48]Syamakrishan *et al.* in preparation. Here in some cases the liquid is replaced by sour rice-gruel (*dhānyāmla*) as it can be made available easily and more importantly in a sterile form when compared to cow's urine (*gomūtra*). This also yielded very good results, suggesting that a formula for an enema (*vastiyoga*) can be regarded as a model and a physician can modify it according to the clinical conditions in which it is administered.

Verse	*Indication*	*VT*	*C*	*Ā*	*V*
1	acute pain (*śūla*)	+	+		+
2	strangury (*ānāha*)	+	+		
3	constipation (*āmavāta*)	+	+		+
4	dropsy (*śotha*)			+	
5	sluggish digestion (*mandāgnitā*)			+	
6	pelvic stiffness (*gṛdhrasī*)			+	+
7	knee-contraction (*jānusaṅkoca*)			+	+
8	muscular rigidity (*saṃstambha*)			+	
9	irregular fever (*viṣamajvara*)			+	+
10	swelling of the hip, thigh and back (*kaṭyūrupṛṣṭhaśotha*)				+
11	persistent torpor of the thigh (*cira-bhavam ūrustambha*)				+
12	impotence (*klaibya*)				+

Table 7.3: *VT*= Vṛnda/Toḍara, *C* = Cakra, *Ā* = *Āyurvedasāra*, *V* = Vaṅgasena

by the decoction of yellow-fruit nightshade, etc. (*vyāghryādikvāthā*).[49]

Time of administration

Vṛnda and Vaṅgasena explain that *vaitaraṇavasti* can be administered to all types of patients.[50] It may even be given after eating, which deviates from the general norm of ad-

[49]Vāgbhaṭa mentions wind-phlegm fever (*vātakaphajvara*), wheezing (*śvāsa*), cough (*kāsa*), catarrh (*pīnasa*), and acute pain (*śūla*) as indications. The *Cikitsāsaṅgraha* and the *Śāraṅgadharasaṃhitā* (Śāstrī 1931: 151) add facial paralysis (*ardita*), lingering fever (*jīrṇajvara*), loss of appetite (*aruci*), loss of voice (*vaisvaryaṃ*), and indigestion (*ajīraṇa*). Govindadāsa adds night fever (*rātrijvara*). Niścalakara reports its high efficacy in old catarrh (*purāṇapīnasa*).

[50]See n. 22 above, verse 190.

ministering non-oily enemas (*nirūhavasti*).[51] It may also be given in the evening. If the strength of the patient is good, then this enema can be given even on empty stomach, although most authorities favour the administration of the Rescue Clyster (*vaitaraṇavasti*) after eating.[52]

Conclusion

In the *Nirukta*, Yāska's ancient work on lexicography and scriptural hermeneutics (*ca.* 5th century BCE), the author says that when the direct seers of the hymns or mantras had passed away, the people approached the gods and asked them about how to fill the void created by the absence of the seers. Then, Yāska answered his own question by saying that etymology (*nirukta*) or reasoning (*tarka*) was transmitted to the people by the gods to fill the void. If the mantras are grasped in the light of the *Nirukta*, then this science is capable of revealing the meaning of the mantras as they were communicated to the original seers.[53] The *Niru-*

---

[51]*Cakradatta* 71.31cd (Sharma 1993: 863): *vaitaraṇaḥ kṣārabastir bhukte cāpi pradīyate|*

[52]*Ratnaprabhāṭīkā* commentary on *Cakradatta* 71.30–31 (Sharma 1993: 863): *atyantaśūlapīdāyāṃ bastidvayam idaṃ bhukte 'pi dīyatā ity āha vaitaraṇa ity ādi| etad āvasthikaṃ vidhānaṃ na tv autsargikaṃ, bhukte nirūhasyeti doṣakartṛtvāt| kin tu bhukte kṣārabastir na punaś carati, vaitaranaḥ punaḥ svasthāvasthāyāṃ pracaraty eva|*
Tattvacandrikāṭīkā commentary, *ibid.* (Bhaṭṭācārya and Bhaṭṭācārya 1933: 891): *atyantaśūlapīdāyāṃ bastidvayam idaṃ bhukte 'pi dīyatā ity āha vaitaraṇa ity ādi| atyantaśūlapīḍāvasthāyām āvasthikam idaṃ vidhānaṃ bodhyaṃ, na tu sārvakālikaṃ, bhukte nirūhasyātidoṣalatvāt| kiṃ tu bhukte kṣāravastir na pracarati, vaitaraṇas tu caraty eva|*

[53]*Nirukta pariśiṣṭa* 13.12 (Sarup 1967: 227): *manuṣyā vā ṛṣiṣūtkrāmatsu devān abruvan| ko na ṛṣir bhaviṣyatīti| tebhya etaṃ tarkam ṛṣiṃ prāyacchan mantrārthacintābhyūham abhyūḷham| tasmād yad eva kiṃcānūcāno 'bhyūhaty ārṣaṃ tad bhavati|* [For the same concept in the main body of the *Nirukta*, cf. section 1.20 (Sarup 1967: text pp. 41–42, tr. p. 20) *sākṣātkṛtadharmāṇa … vedaṃ ca vedāṅgāni ca.* – ed.]

kta provides the missing link and the creative organization of Vedic students, and it is hailed as a sacred teaching that sanctions creative investigation (*ūha-brahma*).[54] Kharanāda noted that when specifics are not mentioned in the texts one must rely on the clinical experience of learned physicians, and use appropriate quantities of drugs after proper assessment of a patient's humours (*doṣa*) and observable variables.[55] By combining these two methods we can design novel paradigms in our research and clinical practice and move forward in new and fruitful directions.

The study of the textual sources of Ayurvedic practice not only helps us to understand the work of indologists, historians, linguists, and philosophers, it also directly benefits our clinical practice and its results. We can move forward in the direction of standardising the *vaitaraṇavasti* by doing rigorous clinical research based on the available textual data.

Further reading

Ācārya, Yādavaśarman Trivikrama (ed.) 1938. *Suśrutasaṃhitā, Suśrutena viracitā, VaidyavaraśrīḌalhaṇācāryaviracitayā Nibandhasaṃgrahākhyavyākhyayā samullasitā, Ācāryopāhvena Trivikramātmajena Yādavaśarmaṇṇā saṃśodhitā.* Mumbayyāṃ: Nirṇayasāgara Mudrāyantrālaye, 3rd edn.

[54]Durga's commentary on the same passage (Bhadkamkar 1942: 1181): *idaṃ niruktaśāstraṃ ūhaḥ brahma yeṣāṃ asti te śabdārthasaṃkateṣv apratibadhyamānā atikramya avidvāṃsaṃ vi-viśeṣataḥ sarvatraiva pratipūjyamānāḥ caranti tve eke ity arthaḥ| evam etasmin mantre asyā udgāhitārthān evoddiśya mantrārthacintābhyūhasya brahmatvaṃ śrūyate|*

[55]Kharaṇāda quoted by Candraṭa, *Cikitsākalikā* 82 (Sharma 1987: 55): *yasmin nirūhe nirdiṣṭāḥ pramāṇaṃ na ca kīrtitam| tasmin doṣādhikaṃ dṛṣṭvā yuktyā saṃvibhajed bhiṣak| madanānāṃ vimṛdyāṃśaṃ kvāthaṃ kṣīrarasādiṣu| śāstraprāptavinyāsaṃ kalpayed guruśikṣayā|*

— 1941. *Maharṣiṇā Punarvasunopadiṣṭā, tacchiṣyeṇāgniveśena praṇītā, CarakaDṛḍhabalābhyāṃ pratisaṃskṛtā Carakasaṃhitā, śrīCakrapāṇidattaviracitayā āyurvedadīpikāvyākhyayā saṃvalitā.* Mumbayyāṃ: Nirṇayasāgara Mudrāyantrālaye, 3rd edn.

Ācārya, Yādavaśarman Trivikrama and Nandakiśora Śarman (eds.) 1939. *Suśrutasaṃhitāyāḥ sūtrasthānam. ŚrīCakrapāṇidattaviracitayā Bhānumatīvyākhyāyā sametam = Sushrut-Sañhitā (Sūtra Sthān) with Bhānumatī Commentary by Chakrapāṇi Datta with introduction by Gaṇanāth Sen*, vol. 1 of *Śrīsvāmi Lakṣmīrāma Nidhi Granthamālā = Shrī Swāmī Lakshmī Rām Trust Series*. Agra: Śyāmasundara Śarman. Printed at the Nirṇayasāgara Press, Bombay.

Bhaṭṭācārya, Āśubodha Vidyābhūṣaṇa and Nityabodha Vidyāratna Bhaṭṭācārya (eds.) 1933. *Cakradatta = Cikitsāsaṃgrahagranthaḥ. MahāmahopādhyāyacarakacaturānanaśrīmacCakrapāṇidattena viracitaḥ. śrīŚivadāsasenaviracitayā Tattvacandrikāsamākhyayā vyākhyayā samalaṅkṛtaḥ.* Kalikātāmahānagaryyāṃ: The editors. Printed at the Vācaspatyayantra.

— 1993. *Cakradatta = Cikitsāsaṃgrahagranthaḥ. MahāmahopādhyāyacarakacaturānanaśrīmacCakrapāṇidattena viracitaḥ. śrīŚivadāsasenaviracitayā Tattvacandrikāsamākhyayā vyākhyayā samalaṅkṛtaḥ*, vol. 14 of *Vidyāvilāsa Āyurveda Granthamālā*. Vārāṇasī: Caukhambhā Oriyanṭāliyā. Page references are to the 1933 edition, Bhaṭṭācārya and Bhaṭṭācārya (1933).

Bhaṭṭācārya , Jīvānanda Vidyāsāgara (ed.) 1893. *Cikitsāsārasaṃgrahaḥ. ŚrīVaṅgasenasaṅkalitaḥ.* Kalikātā: Jīvānanda Vidyāsāgara Bhaṭṭācārya at the Siddheśvarayantra, 2nd edn.

Bhadkamkar, R. G. (ed.) 1942. *The Nirukta of Yāska (With Nighaṇṭu) edited with Durga's Commentary, Vol. II*, vol. 85

of *Bombay Sanskrit and Prakrit Series*. Bombay: R. N. Dandekar for the Dept. Public Instruction, Bombay. V.2 covers chapters 8–12, pariśiṣṭas 13 and 14, and indexes.

Dash, Bhagwan and Lalitesh Kashyap 1980–1992. *[The Āyurveda Saukhyaṃ of the Ṭoḍarānanda]*. Ṭoḍarānanda-Āyurveda Saukhyam Series. New Delhi: Concept Publishing Company. 8 vols., each with a different title.

— 1992. *Five Specialised Therapies of Ayurveda (Pancakarma) based on Ayurveda Saukhyam of Todarananda*, vol. 8 of *Ṭoḍarānanda-Āyurveda Saukhya Series*. New Delhi: Concept Publishing Company. English and Sanskrit.

Devaraj, Therany Lakkannagowda 1972. *Keralīya-pañcakarma-cikitsā-vijñānam*, vol. 65 of *Vidyābhavana Āyurveda granthamālā*. Vārāṇasī: Caukhambā Vidyābhavana, 1st edn. This provides Ārya Vaidyan S. Raghunātha Iyer Śarma's *Keralīya kriyākarma*, with Sanskrit text and Hindi translation by Dr T. L. Devraj .

Jaina, Śaṅkaralāla (ed.) 1904. *Vaṅgasena, Vaṅgasenaviduṣā viracitaḥ. Śāligrāmajīvaiśyaviracitayā bhāṣāṭīkayā samalaṅkṛtaḥ. Śaṅkaralālajainapariśodhitaḥ paripūritaś ca*. Mumbaī: Khemarāja Śrīkṛṣṇadāsa Śreṣṭhinā. Reprinted 1996.

— 1996. *Vaṅgasena, Vaidyakagrantha Vaṅgasenaviduṣā viracitaḥ. Śāligrāmajīvaiśyaviracitayā bhāṣāṭīkayā samalaṅkṛtaḥ. Śaṅkaralālajainapariśodhitaḥ paripūritaś ca*. Mumbaī: Khemarāja Śrīkṛṣṇadāsa Śreṣṭhinā. Reprint of 1904 edition.

Kṛṣṇanvaidyan, C. (ed.) 1988. *Vastipradīpaṃ by Pāṇavaḷḷi*. C. K. Raghavan Vaidyan at C. K. V. Hospital, Panavally: C. K. Raghavan Vaidyan, 2nd edn. First published 10/10/1108 Kollaṃ Era.

Keśavanvaidyan, Manakoḍaṃ K. (ed.) 1993. *Pañcakarma athavā śodhanacikitsā*. Cheratala: M. K. Ravindran Vaidyan, 2nd edn. First edition 1949.

Kumṭe, Aṇṇā Moreśvara, Kṛṣṇaśāstrī Navare, and Hariśāstrī Parādkar (eds.) 1995. *Aṣṭāṅgahṛdayam, śrīmadvāgbhaṭaviracitam, śrīmadaruṇadattaviracitayā 'sarvāṅgasundaryākhyā' vyākhyayā hemādripraṇītayā 'āyurvedarasāyanāhvayā' ṭīkayā ca samullasitam*, vol. 4 of *Krishnadas Ayurveda Series*. Vārāṇasī: Krishnadas Academy. Cited from the 2002 reprint.

Menon, Poyyayil Putiyedathu Raman (ed.) 1929/1930. *Śrī śirassekādi vidhi with Bhāvaprabodhinī Malayalam commentary*. Cranganore: Raman Menon. Date of publication given as 1105 ME.

Meulenbeld, Gerrit Jan 1999–2002. *A History of Indian Medical Literature*, vol. XV of *Groningen Oriental Studies*. Groningen: E. Forsten. 5v.

Mooss, Dhanwantharidas C. N. Narayanam (ed.) 1940. *The Ashtangahridaya composed by Vahatacharya, with the commentary of Sreedasapandita, Part I*, vol. 4 of *Sri Chithra Ayurveda Series*. Trivandrum: Government Press.

Mooss, N. S. 1983. *Ayurvedic treatments of Kerala*, vol. E-5 of *Vaidyasarathy Series*. Kottayam: Vaidyasarathy Press, 3rd edn.

Muthuswami, N. E. (ed.) 1976. *Rasavaiśeṣikasūtra, Bhadanta Nāgārjunaviracitam, Narasiṃhakṛtabhāṣyopetam*, vol. 2 of *Kerala Government Ayurvedic Publication Series*. Trivandrum: Govt. Ayurveda College.

Nīlakaṇṭhaśarma, T. and Yādavaśarman Trivikrama Ācārya (eds.) 1913. *Dhārākalpa*. Bombay: Yādavaśarman Trivikrama Ācārya.

Nambiyār Vaidyar, P. Cāttukkuṭṭi (ed.) 1960. *Yogāmṛtaṃ: Saṃpūrṇa Yogāmṛtaṃ*. Kannur: Srisadan Ayurveda Oushadhasala.

Pādhye, Haṇamantaśāstrī (ed.) 1894. *Vṛndamādhavāparanāmakasiddhayoga, with Śrīkaṇṭhadatta's commentary*, vol. 27

of *Ānandāśrama Sanskrit Series*. Poona: Ānandāśrama Press.

Raghavan, V., K. Kunjunni Raja, C. S. Sundaram, N. Veezhinathan, N. Gangadharan, *et al.* 1949–. *New Catalogus Catalogorum, an Alphabetical Register of Sanskrit and Allied Works and Authors*. Madras University Sanskrit Series. Madras: University of Madras.

Raghunatha Iyer, Aryavaidyan S. 1972. *Keralīya pañcakarma vijñānaṃ*. Varanasi: Chowkhambha Vidyabhavan.

Rama Rao, B. 2005. *Sanskrit Medical Manuscripts in India*. Delhi: CCRAS.

Rāya, Rāma Kumāra (ed.) 1983. *Baṅgasena-saṃhitā (Cikitsāsāra saṃgraha). Hindī vyākhyākāra Rājīva Kumāra Rāya*, vol. 1 of *Dhanvantari Granthamālā*. Vārāṇasī: Prācya Prakāśana, 1st edn.

van Rheede, Henricus 1678–1703. *Hortus Indicus Malabaricus....* Amstelaedami: Joannis van Someren and Joannis van Dyck. 12v.

Sarup, Lakshman 1967. *The Nighaṇṭu and The Nirukta, The Oldest Indian Treatise on Etymology, Philology, and Sementics [sic]*. Delhi, Varanasi, Patna: Motilal Banarsidass.

Sasikumar, V. K., P. Sankarankutty, and M. R. Vasudevan Namboodiri (eds.) 1991. *A Study of Low Back Ache and its Management with Vaitaraṇavasti*. Thiruvananthapuram: Government Ayurveda College.

Śāstrī, Paraśurāma (ed.) 1931. *DāmodarasūnuŚārṅgadharācāryaviracitā Śārṅgadharasaṃhitā. BhiṣagvarĀḍhamallaviracitadīpikāKāśīrāmavaidyaviracitagūḍhārthadīpikābhyāṃ, ṭīkābhyāṃ, saṃvalitā*. Muṃbai: Nirṇayasāgara Press, 2nd edn. References are to the 1983 reprint from Caukhambha Sanskrit Series Office, Varanasi.

Sharma, Priya Vrat 1975. *Āyurved kā Vaijñānik Itihās*, vol. 1 of *Jayakṛṣṇadāsa Āyurveda Granthamālā*. Vārāṇasī:

Caukhambā Orientalia. Reference is to the 2004 reprint.

Sharma, Priya Vrat (ed.) 1987. *Tīsaṭācāryakṛtā Cikitsā-kalikā tadātmaja-śrīCandraṭapraṇītayā saṃskṛtavyākhyayā saṃvalitā, Aṅglabhāṣā-vyākhyātā tathā pariṣkartā ācārya Priyavrata Śarmā*. Vārāṇasī: Caukhambā Surabhāratī Prakāśana.

— 1993. *Cakradatta or Cikitsāsaṅgraha of Cakrapāṇidatta with Ratnaprabhāṭīkā by Mahāmahopādhyāya Śri Niścalakara*. Jaipur: Swami Jayaramadas Ramprakash Trust, 1st edn.

Syamakrishan, G. *et al*. in preparation. "A Critical Appraisal of Evidence-based Medicine: Some Ethical Considerations with Special Reference to Effect of Vaitaraṇavasti in Low Back Ache."

Tivārī, Premavatī (ed.) 2007. *Vṛndamādhava athavā Siddha yoga = Vṛndamādhava or Siddha Yoga: the First Treatise of Āyurveda on Treatment*, vol. 18 of *Haridas Ayurveda Series*. Varanasi: Chaukhambha Visvabharati, 1st edn. 2v.

8

K. G. Zysk
and
T. Yamashita

Jajjaṭa's *Nirantarapadavyākhyā* on the *Carakasaṃhitā*, *Cikitsāsthāna* 2.1.1-4ab

Introduction

The *Nirantarapadavyākhyā* by Jajjaṭa (or Jejjaṭa) is one of the earliest and, therefore, one of the most important commentaries on the *Carakasaṃhitā*.[1] This commentary is incomplete, but sufficient portions survive to allow a study of the earliest form of medical commentary in India. The extant portions of this commentary are large sections of the Cikitsāsthāna and part of the Kalpasthāna and Siddhisthāna of the *Carakasaṃhitā*. The text of Jajjaṭa has never been critically edited. Our study is based on several copies of a lost palm-leaf manuscript in Malayalam script and the printed edition by Haridatta Śāstrin in 1941.[2]

Jajjaṭa's descriptive method follows that of a traditional commentarial style (*ṭīkā*) in Sanskrit with a specialization in Ayurvedic terminology and concepts. A principal aim of the commentator is the establishment of the correct reading of the original (*mūla*) text, which in places varies from the printed editions of the *Carakasaṃhitā* extant today. This may

[1]For a full description of Jajjaṭa's commentary, see Zysk 2009.
[2]Haridatta Śāstrin 1941.

point to the existence of a different recension of the *Carakasaṃhitā*, that was known to Jajjaṭa, and suggest that the text of the *Carakasaṃhitā* was still in the process of evolution at the time.

In this chapter, we present a sample of the edition and translation of Jajjaṭa's *Nirantarapadavyākhyā* on the *Carakasaṃhitā Cikitsāsthāna* 2.1.1–4ab.[3]

Notes

Manuscripts and printed editions

THE *NIRANTARAPADAVYĀKHYĀ* BY JAJJAṬA

M^m^ Malayalam manuscript in Madras/Chennai (1919–1920).
R 2983 in the Government Oriental Manuscripts Library in Madras/Chennai. It is a transcription in modern Malayalam script on 254 folia begun in the latter part of 1919 and completed in 1920. Its source was a palm-leaf manuscript owed by M. R. Ry. Vaidyan Variyar, who resided at Trippunithura in what was then called Cochin State. The text is incomplete, covering the commentary to parts of the *Cikitsāsthāna*, *Kalpasthāna* and *Siddhisthāna* of the *Carakasaṃhitā*.

T^d^ Devanāgarī manuscript in Trivandrum (1930).
The Nāgarī copy, occurring in three parts, corresponds to manuscript no. T. 850 in the collection of

[3]For the edition, we use copies of manuscripts made available to us by Dominik Wujastyk and also – under an Agreement of Cooperation and Agreement for Use of Manuscript Materials – by the research project "Philosophy and Medicine in Early Classical India II" (FWF project P19866) (August 1, 2007 – November 30, 2010) directed by Prof. Dr Karin Preisendanz and conducted at the Institute for South Asian, Tibetan and Buddhist Studies at the University of Vienna. We would like to extend our gratitude to Prof. Dr Karin Preisendanz and Dr Philipp Maas.

the University of Trivandum Library and to no. 835 in the collection of the Curator's Office Library, Trivandrum. The two numbers refer to the same manuscript. According to K. Mahādeva Śāstrin, the owner of the copy was a certain Nārāyaṇa Mūss Mūttatu, from Idayindathu in British Cochin.[4] This is confirmed by the title pages of the copy. Although the pages are numbered consecutively from 1–307, the manuscript is divided into three parts and appears to be by two different scribes. The copy was ultimately completed in 1930.

J^{d} Devanāgarī manuscript in Jamnagar (1945?).
The Nāgarī copy, No. 78, GAS 115 in Gujarat Ayurved University, Jamnagar. This manuscript is written on modern yellow paper, pages 1–295 being bound as a notebook, dimensions 20.5×33.5 cm. On the last page is written "copied by C. N. Subramanya Sastry, 1-3-45 and compared 6-3-45". The date is presumably 1945. The text is written in black ink and written over in red ink in places.

Ś^{e} Printed edition edited by Haridatta Śāstrin (1941).
There is only one printed edition, that published in 1941.[5] It was made by Haridatta Śāstrin and was based on the Malayalam transcript (the abovementioned **M^{m}**), R 2983 in the Government Oriental Manuscript Library, Madras. Haridatta Śāstrin explains that the original is a palm-leaf manuscript and that the gaps in the text were filled in by his own hand which, he says, was guided by the context of the subject-matter surrounding the missing parts. Although Haridatta Śāstrin's attempt to

---

[4]Śāstrin 1939: v. 5, pp. 1817–18; Kunjan Pillai 1957: v. 1, p. 216.

[5]Haridatta Śāstrin 1941.

provide clarity and consistency is commendable, at times his eagerness crosses the boundary of what is considered acceptable by modern editors.

The *Carakasaṃhitā*

Ch[d] Devanāgarī manuscript.
Lal Chand Research Library, Dayanand Anglo-Vedic College, Chandigarh, MS 2315.

J2[d] Devanāgarī manuscript.
Raghunath Temple Library of His Highness the Maharaja of Jammu and Kashmir, Jammu, MS 3209.

V[e] Printed Edition.
Edited by Jīvānanda Vidyāsāgara Bhaṭṭācāryya, and printed at the Sarasvati Press, Calcutta, in 1877 (Bhaṭṭācāryya 1877).

G[e] Printed Edition.
Edited by Gaṅgāviṣṇu Śrīkṛṣṇadāsa and printed at the Lakṣmīveṅkaṭeśvara Steam Press in 1932 (Gaṅgāviṣṇu Śrīkṛṣṇadāsa 1932) .

T[e] Printed Edition.
Edited by Yādava Trivikrama Ācārya, 3rd edition, Bombay: Nirṇaya-sāgar Press, 1941 (Ācārya 1941). Fourth edition, New Delhi: Munshiram Manoharlal Publishers, 1981.

Text

bold phrases of the *Carakasaṃhitā* which are commented upon at that place (*lemmata*)

bold italic
quotations from elsewhere in the *Carakasaṃhitā*

italic quotations from texts other than the *Carakasaṃhitā*

commas and full stops
are used for punctuation, not *daṇḍa*s

numbering
: of the verses and passages of the *Carakasaṃhitā* is based on those given in T^e

APPARATUS (NUMBERED BEGINNING AT THE TOP)

Apparatus 1
: the page and line numbers of the manuscripts and the printed edition

Apparatus 2
: variants found in the manuscripts and the printed edition

Apparatus 3
: breaks or *daṇḍa*s in the manuscripts and the printed edition (For the sake of simplicity, only commas and full stops are used, not *daṇḍas*. $\mathbf{M}^{\mathbf{m}}$ basically does not show any breaks)

Apparatus 4 (if present)
: quotations from the *Carakasaṃhitā*

Apparatus 5 (if present)
: quotations from the other Ayurvedic texts than the *Carakasaṃhitā*

Apparatus 6 (if present)
: quotations from the other texts than the Ayurvedic texts

SIGNS

[ ]	insertion (the number of verse, etc.) by the editor
[·]	illegible portion
[–]	illegible portion by the page bounding (only in $\mathbf{J2}^{d}$)
⟨···⟩	gap or missing portion indicated by the scribe by a space with or without ··· dots. The space indicated is approximately proportional to the space in the manuscript, according to three categories: small

⟨·⟩, middle ⟨· · ·⟩, and large ⟨· · · · · ·⟩. Spaces are not estimated precisely.

⟨~~a~~⟩ text deleted, probably by the scribe

⟨⟩ corrective insertion (interlinear or marginal), probably made by the same scribe

⟨^{2}~~a~~⟩ text deleted by a second hand

⟨^{2} ⟩ a corrective insertion (interlinear or in margin), probably added by a second hand

⟨*ac*⟩ *ante correctionem* = before correction

⟨^{2}*pc*⟩ *post correctionem* = after correction, probably by a second hand

n_ the underscore indicates a *virāma* sign, if it needs to be indicated (especially in Apparatus 3)

Abbreviations

AHS *Aṣṭāṅgahṛdayasaṃhitā* (Kuṃṭe *et al.* 1902; seventh edition, *idem* 1982)

AS *Aṣṭāṅgasaṃgraha* (Āṭhavale 1980).

BauDhS *Baudhāyana Dharmasūtra* (Bhaṭṭācāryya 1876)

Ci *Cikitsāsthāna*

CS *Carakasaṃhitā*

em. emendation

MDh *Mānava Dharmaśāstra* or *Manu Smṛti* (Nene 1970)

om. omission

Śā *Śārīrasthāna*

ŚB *Śatapatha Brāhmaṇa* (Weber 1964)

ŚKD *Śabdakalpadruma* (Rādhākānta 1876)

Sū *Sūtrasthāna*

TS *Taittirīya Saṃhitā* (Āgāśe and Taḷekara 1959–1978)

Utt *Uttaratantra* or *Uttarasthāna*

Edition

svasthasyorjaskaraṃ yat tu tad vṛṣyaṃ tad rasāyanam. ity uktatvād rasāyanaṃ vājīkaraṇam api tad bhavati. na tu tadātva eva, yathā vājīkaraṇaṃ tasya prayojanam abhidhāsyati. atraivaitad anantaraṃ vājīkaraṇārambhaḥ.

tac ca caturṣv api pādeṣv eka evādhyāyaḥ, dvayam apy etad adhyāya-dvayam ucyata iti.

tasmāt saṃyogaśaramūlādīnām ekādhyāyatvād eka eva saṃbandho 'tra ca saṃyogaśaramūlīye vājīkaraṇaprayojanādi sarvam ucyata iti.

tasmāt saṃyogaḥ śaramūlādīnāṃ yasmin pāde vidyate, taṃ saṃyoga-śaramūlīyaṃ vājīkaraṇapādam.

---

1 svasthasyorjaskaraṃ] M^m p.23, *l*.1; J^d p.16, *l*.1; T^d p.21, *l*.1; $Ś^e$ p.838, *l*.6 **10 vājīkaraṇapādam**] M^m p.23, *l*.9; J^d p.16, *l*.8; T^d p.21, *l*.10; $Ś^e$ p.838, *l*.29

---

*At the beginning of this quarter, athātaḥ saṃyogaśaramūlīyaṃ vājīkaraṇapādaṃ vyākhyāsyāmaḥ ‖1‖ iti ha smāha bhagavān ātreyaḥ ‖2‖ $Ś^e$; *om.* $M^mJ^dT^d$
2 tad] J^d; tat M^m; taṃ tad T^d; sad $Ś^e$ **3 atraivaitad**] $Ś^e$; atravatad M^m; atraiva. tad T^d; atraiva tad J^d **7 saṃbandho 'tra**] $J^dT^dŚ^e$; saṃbandhotra M^m **9 taṃ**] $M^mJ^dŚ^e$; *om.* T^d

---

2 bhavati.] J^dT^d; bhavati $Ś^e$ ❁ **eva,**] $T^dŚ^e$; eva[-]thā J^d **3 abhidhāsyati.**] $Ś^e$; abhidhāsyaty J^dT^d **5 evādhyāyaḥ,**] evādhyāyaḥ $J^dŚ^e$; evādhyā<· · ·> T^d **6 ucyata iti.**] T^d; ucyata iti M^m; ucyate. iti. J^d; ucyate iti. $Ś^e$ **8 ucyata iti.**] $T^dŚ^e$; ucyate iti M^m; ucyate. iti J^d **9 vidyate,**] J^dT^d; vidyate $Ś^e$ **10 vājīkaraṇapādam.**] $J^dŚ^e$; vājīkaraṇapādaṃ T^d

---

*At the beginning of this quarter, athātaḥ saṃyogaśaramūlīyaṃ vājīkaraṇapādaṃ vyākhyāsyāmaḥ ‖1‖ iti ha smāha bhagavān ātreyaḥ ‖2‖ $Ś^eT^e$; athātaḥ saṃprayogaśaramūlīyaṃ vājīkaraṇapādaṃ vyākhyāsyāmaḥ | iti ha smāha bhagavān ātreyaḥ ‖ G^e; athātaḥ saṃprayogaśaramūlīyaṃ vājīkaraṇapādaṃ vyākhyāsyāmaḥ | V^e; ataḥ saṃprayogaśaramūlīyaṃ vājīkaraṇapādaṃ vyākhyāsyāmaḥ ‖ $J2^d$; athāttaḥ saṃprayośaramūlīyavājīkaraṇapādaṃ vyākhyāsyāmaḥ ‖ Ch^d
1 svasthasyorjaskaraṃ ... rasāyanam] CS Ci 1.1.5cd $Ś^eT^eG^e$(4cd) V^e; svasthasyojaskaraṃ ... rasāyanaṃ $J2^d$; svasthāsyojaskaraṃ ... vṛṣyat ... Ch^d

vājīkaraṇam anv icchet puruṣo nityam ātmavān. [3ab] ityādi vājīvāśvasadharmā yena kriyate taṃ vājīkaraṇaṃ hi. ***vājīvātibalo yena yāty apratihataḥ striyaḥ.*** iti. kuto nu rasāyanāt tasya hi samupacitadhātoḥ pradhānadhātuparikṣayo mā bhūd iti. anuśabdo bahuṣv apy artheṣu< · · · >paścād vacanaṃ yat sevyam, maithunād anu, paścād ity arthaḥ. puruṣagrahaṇaṃ bālātyantavr̥ddhanirāsārtham. vakṣyati,

atibālo hy asaṃpūrṇasarvadhātuḥ striyo vrajan.
upatapyeta sahasā taṭākam iva nirjalam.
śuṣkaṃ rūkṣaṃ yathā kāṣṭhaṃ jantujagdhaṃ vijarjaram.

---

11 vājīvāśvasadharmā] (Ś^{e} p.839, *l.*1)vājīvāśvasadharmā **17 bālātyanta**] bālā(T^{d} p.22, *l.*1)tyanta

---

12 yena] M^{m}J^{d}Ś^{e}; yona T^{d} ❀ **vājīkaraṇaṃ hi**] M^{m}J^{d}Ś^{e}; vājīkara<·>hi T^{d} **13 -hataḥ striyaḥ**] Ś^{e}; hataḥ stri[·]ḥ M^{m}; hataḥ stri⟨^{2}~~śca~~⟩⟨^{2}ya⟩ḥ J^{d}; hatastraya T^{d} ❀ **kuto nu**] M^{m}T^{d}Ś^{e}; kuto 'nu J^{d} **15 artheṣu< · · · >paścād**] M^{m}J^{d}; atve<·>paścād T^{d}; artheṣu (prayujyate. atra tu) paścād Ś^{e} *em.* ❀ **sevyam maithunād**] M^{m}J^{d}Ś^{e}; sevyate<·>nād T^{d} **18 atibālo**] M^{m}J^{d}Ś^{e}; atibalo T^{d} ❀ **-pūrṇasarvadhātuḥ**] pūrṇa(sarva)dhātuḥ Ś^{e} *em.* ; pūrṇadhātuḥ M^{m}; pūrṇadhātu T^{d}; pūrṇadhā[-] J^{d} **19 upatapyeta...taṭākam**] Ś^{e}; upatapyeta ... taḍākam M^{m}J^{d}; upa<·>taṭākam T^{d} **20 śuṣkaṃ**] J^{d}T^{d}Ś^{e}; śūṣkaṃ M^{m}

---

13 iti.] J^{d}T^{d}; iti Ś^{e} **14 iti.**] ity J^{d}T^{d}Ś^{e} **15 sevyam,**] sevyaṃ J^{d}Ś^{e}; sevyate T^{d} **16 anu,**] anu M^{m}J^{d}T^{d}Ś^{e} **17 vakṣyati,**] Ś^{e}; vakṣyaty J^{d}T^{d}

11 vājīkaraṇam ... ātmavān] CS Ci 2.1.3ab T^{e}V^{e}G^{e}J2^{d}Ch^{d} **13 vājīvātibalo ... striyaḥ**] CS Ci 1.1.9cd T^{e}V^{e}G^{e}; ... apratihatastriyaḥ J2^{d}; ... apratihatāḥ striyaḥ Ch^{d} **18 atibālo ... vrajan**] CS Ci 2.4.41ab V^{e}G^{e}J2^{d}Ch^{d}; ... asaṃpūrṇasarvadhātuḥ striyaṃ vrajan T^{e} **19 upatapyeta ... nirjalam**] CS Ci 2.4.41cd ... taḍāgam iva kājalam V^{e}G^{e}; ... taḍākam iva kājalam J^{d}Ch^{d}; upaśuṣyeta sahasā taḍāgam iva kājalam T^{e} **20 śuṣkaṃ ... vijarjaram**] CS Ci 2.4.42ab T^{e}; śuṣkavr̥kṣaṃ yathā kāṣṭhaṃ jantudagdhaṃ vijarjaram V^{e}J2^{d}Ch^{d}; śuṣkarūkṣaṃ ... G^{e}

---

11 vājīkaraṇam ... ātmavān] AHS Utt 40.1ab=AS Utt 50.2ab vājīkaraṇam anv icchet satataṃ viṣayī pumān **13 vājīvātibalo ... striyaḥ**] AHS Utt 40.2cd=AS Utt 50.3ab ... apratihato 'ṅganāḥ **18 atibālo ... vrajan**] AS Sū 9.59ab ... striyaṃ vrajan **19 upatapyeta ... nirjalam**] AS Sū 9.59cd ... kājalam **20 śuṣkaṃ ... vijarjaram**] AS Sū 9.60ab

spṛṣṭam āśu viśīryeta tathā vṛddhaḥ striyo vrajan.

na punaḥ strīṣaṇḍavyudāsārtham, teṣāṃ vājīkaraṇāprāpteḥ. nityagrahaṇaṃ sadā sevanaṃ jñāpayati. yathā rasāyanaṃ prayuktaṃ sarvadhātūnāṃ puṣṭim ādadhāti, naivaṃ vājīkaraṇam. tad dhi satatam upayujyamānam āhāravac chukradhātuvṛddhim ādadhātīti. ātmavadgrahaṇena dhṛtim ato 'nujñāṃ vidadhāti. ya eva dhṛtyā niyantuṃ paradārādibhyaḥ śaknoti sa evādhikriyate, na paśur ivāgamyāgamana< · · · >m ullaṅghya pravartate. sarvadā jitendriyasyādhikāreṇa prayojanāyāha,

yadā yat tau hi dharmārthau prītiś ca yaśa eva ca. [3cd]
putrasyāyatanaṃ hy etad guṇāś caite sutāśrayāḥ. [4ab] iti.

---

22 -karaṇāprāpteḥ] karaṇāprā(M^{m} p.24, *l.*1)pteḥ **30 yadā]** (J^{d} p.17, *l.*1)yadā

---

jantujagdhaṃ] M^{m}J^{d}Ś^{e}; jantujaḍaṃ T^{d} ❁ **vijarjaram]** J^{d}Ś^{e}; vijarjjaraṃ M^{m}; vijaraṃ T^{d}

21 spṛṣṭam] M^{m}J^{d}Ś^{e}; praṣṭam T^{d} ❁ **vṛddhaḥ striyo]** M^{m}J^{d}Ś^{e}; vṛddhastriyo T^{d} **22 -vyudāsārtham ... 23 jñāpayati]** M^{m}J^{d}Ś^{e}; vyuda<·>jñāpayati T^{d} **23 yathā]** M^{m}J^{d}Ś^{e}; tathā T^{d} **24 -dhātūnāṃ]** M^{m}Ś^{e}; dh[-]tūnāṃ J^{d}; bhūtānāṃ T^{d} **25 āhāravac]** M^{m}J^{d}T^{d}; ahāravac Ś^{e} ❁ **chukradhātu]** Ś^{e}; chukladhātu M^{m}J^{d}; cha<·>tu T^{d} **26 ato 'nujñāṃ]** T^{d}Ś^{e}; atonujñāṃ M^{m}; at[-] 'nujñāṃ J^{d} **27 ivāgamyāgamana< · · · >m]** M^{m}J^{d}; ivāgamyā<·>gam T^{d}; ivāgamyāgamana(niṣedhaśāstra)m Ś^{e} *em.* **28 jitendriyasyādhikāreṇa]** Ś^{e}; jitendriyasyādhikāran na M^{m}; jitendriyasyādhikāraṃ na J^{d}; jitendriyasyādhikāraṇa T^{d} **30 yadā yat tau]** M^{m}J^{d}T^{d}; yadā 'yat tau Ś^{e} **31 putrasyāyatanaṃ]** T^{e}V^{e}G^{e}J2^{d}Ch^{d}; putrasya yatanaṃ M^{m}J^{d}Ś^{e}; putravyāyatanaṃ T^{d} **etad]** J^{d}; etat M^{m}Ś^{e}; ekaṃ T^{d} ❁ **caite sutāśrayāḥ]** J^{d}Ś^{e}; caite sutāśrayā M^{m}; cai< · · · > T^{d} ❁ **iti...32 sutāśrayā]** J^{d} ⟨^{2}*pc*⟩; *om.* J^{d} ⟨*ac*⟩

---

22 -vyudāsārtham,] J^{d}; vyudāsārthaṃ Ś^{e}; vyuda<·> T^{d} ❁ **-karaṇāprāpteḥ.]** Ś^{e}; karaṇāprāpteḥ J^{d}; *lacuna* T^{d} **23 yathā]** Ś^{e}; yathā. J^{d}; tathā T^{d} **25 ādadhātīti.]** Ś^{e}; ādadhātīti J^{d}; ādadhātīty T^{d} **27 śaknoti]** T^{d}Ś^{e}; śaknoti. J^{d} **29 prayojanāyāha,]** T^{d}Ś^{e}; prayojanāyāh[-] J^{d} **31 sutāśrayāḥ.]** J^{d}; *lacuna* T^{d} ; sutāśrayāḥ Ś^{e} ❁ **iti.]** Ś^{e}; ⟨^{2}iti⟩ J^{d}; < · · · >. T^{d}

---

21 spṛṣṭam ... vrajan] CS Ci 2.4.42cd T^{e}G^{e}; ... vṛddhastriyo ... V^{e}J2^{d}Ch^{d} **30 yadā ... ca^{2}]** CS Ci 2.1.3cd tadā ... T^{e}V^{e}G^{e}J2^{d}Ch^{d} **31 putrasyāyatanaṃ ... sutāśrayāḥ]** CS Ci 2.1.4ab T^{e}V^{e}G^{e}J2^{d}Ch^{d}

---

21 spṛṣṭam ... vrajan] AS Sū 9.60cd ... striyaṃ vrajan

dharmārthayaśaḥprītiputrāptayaḥ prayojanam iti. kathaṃ sutāśrayā dharmādayaḥ ucyate, dharmaḥ putrotpādanāt. tathā ca śrutiḥ, *brāhmaṇas tribhir ṛṇair ṛṇavān bhavati. agnihotreṇa devānām, brahmacaryeṇa ṛṣīṇām, prajayā pitṝṇām, tathā nāputrasya loko 'sti.* iti. *sarve vai paśavo vidur ye na te mātary api mithunaṃ caranti.* iti. athavā< · · · >pitarau dharmaṃ kārayati. vittaṃ cānyato 'py arjayitvā prayacchati. prītiś cābhimānikī putradarśanāt. āha ca vyāsabhaṭṭārakaḥ, *putrajanmaviyogābhyāṃ na paraṃ sukhaduḥkhayoḥ.* iti. yaś ca pitroḥ pratanoti, satputratvāt. ete ca guṇāḥ putrāśrayāḥ. tasmād **vājīkaraṇam anv icched** [3a] iti yuktam. pravartakaṃ ca dharmaṃ svargaprāptilakṣaṇam āśritya tad ucyate. yan

---

34 devānām] (T^{d} p.23, *l.*1)devānāṃ **40 satputratvāt**] (M^{m} p.25, *l.*1)satputratvād

---

32 -yaśaḥ-] M^{m}T^{d}Ś^{e}; yaśāḥ J^{d} ❀ **-prīti-**] T^{d}; kīrti M^{m}J^{d}Ś^{e} ❀ **-putrāptayaḥ**] M^{m}Ś^{e}; putrān āptayaḥ J^{d}; putrāptāptayaḥ T^{d} ❀ **sutāśrayā**] M^{m}Ś^{e}; sutāśraya J^{d}; sutāśrayāḥ T^{d} **33 dharmādayaḥ**] M^{m}Ś^{e}; dharmā⟨~~śrayāḥ~~⟩⟨dayaḥ⟩ J^{d}; dharmādaya T^{d} ❀ **dharmaḥ**] T^{d}Ś^{e}; dharmaṃ M^{m}J^{d} ❀ **ca**] M^{m}J^{d}Ś^{e}; hi T^{d} **34 brāhmaṇas**] M^{m}Ś^{e}; bhrāhmarṇais J^{d}; jāyamāno brāhmaṇas T^{d} ❀ **ṛṇair**] M^{m}; ⟨^{2}ṛṇair⟩ J^{d}; ṛṇaiḥ T^{d}; (ṛ)nair Ś^{e} *em.* ❀ **ṛṇavān bhavati**] Ś^{e}; ṛṇavān< · · · > M^{m}J^{d}; ṛṇa< · > T^{d} **36 vai**] M^{m}J^{d}T^{d}; *om.* Ś^{e} **37 athavā< · · · >pitarau**] M^{m}J^{d}; athavā< · >pitarau T^{d}; athavā (suto hi) pitarau Ś^{e} *em.* ❀ **cānyato 'py**] T^{d}Ś^{e}; cānyatopy M^{m}J^{d} ❀ **arjayitvā**] Ś^{e}; ārjjayitvā M^{m}; ārjayitvā J^{d}T^{d} **38 vyāsabhaṭṭārakaḥ**] M^{m}T^{d}Ś^{e}; vyāsabhaṭṭā⟨^{2}rakaḥ⟩ J^{d} **40 pitroḥ**] M^{m}J^{d}Ś^{e}; pitrau T^{d} ❀ **ete ca guṇāḥ**] M^{m}J^{d}Ś^{e}; alpaguṇāḥ T^{d} **42 ucyate**] M^{m}J^{d}Ś^{e}; ucyante T^{d} ❀ **yan**] M^{m}J^{d}Ś^{e}; kan T^{d}

---

32 iti.] T^{d}Ś^{e}; iti J^{d} **33 putrotpādanāt.**] J^{d}Ś^{e}; putrotpādanāt_ M^{m}; putrotpādanāt T^{d} **34 bhavati.**] Ś^{e}; *lacuna* M^{m}J^{d}T^{d} ❀ **devānām,**] Ś^{e}; devānāṃ J^{d}T^{d} **35 ṛṣīṇām,**] Ś^{e}; ṛṣīṇāṃ J^{d}T^{d} ❀ **pitṝṇām,**] Ś^{e}J^{d}; pitṝṇāṃ T^{d} ❀ **loko 'sti. iti.**] loko 'sti iti J^{d}; loko 'stīti T^{d}; loko 'stīti. Ś^{e} **36 caranti. iti.**] caratīti. J^{d}; carantīty T^{d}; carantīti. Ś^{e} **37 kārayati.**] J^{d}T^{d}; kārayati Ś^{e} **38 putradarśanāt.**] Ś^{e}; putradarśanād J^{d}T^{d} **40 pratanoti,**] T^{d}; pratanoti J^{d}Ś^{e} ❀ **satputratvāt.**] satputratvād J^{d}T^{d}Ś^{e} ❀ **putrāśrayāḥ.**] J^{d}Ś^{e}; putrāśrayās T^{d} **41 yuktam.**] J^{d}T^{d}; yuktaṃ Ś^{e} **42 ucyate.**] J^{d}; ucyate Ś^{e}; ucyante. T^{d}

---

34 brāhmaṇas ... 35 'sti] Cf. TS 6.3.10.5; also ŚB 1.7.2.1-6 and ŚKD 1.284; BauDhS 2.6.11.33-34 (cf. 2.9.16.7) **39 putrajanmaviyogābhyāṃ ... sukha**] The source is unidentified.

nivr̥ttikr̥te hi sa upadeśaḥ, ***kośakāro yathā hy aṃśūn upādatte vadhapradān. tathāgnikalpān arthān jño jñātvā tebhyo nivartate.*** iti. naiḥśreyasikaṃ dharmam āśritya brahmacaryopadeśaḥ. ayaṃ cābhyudayikam iti, na parasparavirodhāśaṅketi. tatraitat syāt, ***traya upaṣṭambhakā bhavanty āhāraḥ svapno brahmacaryam.*** iti. ***ebhir upaṣṭabdham*** ity āder upadeśāt, katham atra strīniṣevaṇam abhihitam. yathā, ***ebhis tribhir yuktiyuktair upaṣṭabdhaṃ śarīraṃ bhavati.*** iti. śukravidhāraṇe ca doṣābhidhānam, ***śukraveganigrahaṇaṃ ṣāṇḍya-***

51 ca] (T^{d} p.24, *l*.1)ca

44 vadhapradān] M^{m}J^{d}Ś^{e}; vadhapradāt T^{d} **45 arthān**] J^{d}Ś^{e}M^{m}; anarthān T^{d} **46 naiḥśreyasikaṃ**] Ś^{e}; naiśreyasikaṃ M^{m}J^{d}T^{d} ❁ **dharmam ... brahmacaryopadeśaḥ**] M^{m}J^{d}Ś^{e}; dharma< · >padeśaḥ T^{d} **47 -virodhāśaṅketi**] M^{m}J^{d}T^{d}; virodhaprasaktir iti Ś^{e} **48 upaṣṭambhakā**] M^{m}J^{d}Ś^{e}; uṣapastaṃbhā T^{d} ❁ **iti**] M^{m}J^{d}Ś^{e}; *om.* T^{d} **49 strīniṣevaṇam**] M^{m}J^{d}Ś^{e}; < · >ṣevaṇam T^{d} **51 śukra-**] M^{m}J^{d}Ś^{e}; śutra T^{d} ❁ **śukravega-**]

45 nivartate. iti.] Ś^{e}; nivartata iti J^{d}; nivartata iti. T^{d} **46 brahmacaryopadeśaḥ.**] J^{d}Ś^{e}; < · >padeśaḥ. T^{d} **47 iti,**] T^{d}; iti J^{d}Ś^{e} ❁ **-virodhāśaṅketi.**] T^{d}; virodhāśaṅketi M^{m}J^{d}; virodhaprasaktir iti. Ś^{e} **48 iti.**] J^{d}Ś^{e}; *om.* T^{d} **49 upadeśāt,**] T^{d}; upadeśāt J^{d}Ś^{e} **50 yathā, ebhis**] yathā ebhis J^{d}T^{d}Ś^{e} ❁ **bhavati. iti.**] bhavatīti J^{d}T^{d}; bhavatīti. Ś^{e} **51 ṣāṇḍyakarāṇām.**] Ś^{e}; ṣāṇḍyakaraṇaṃ J^{d}; ṣaṇḍyakarāṇāṃ T^{d}

44 kośakāro ... vadhapradān] CS Śā 1.96ab V^{e}; koṣakāro ... T^{e}G^{e}; ... vadapradān J2^{d}; ... vadhāvahān Ch^{d} **45 tathāgnikalpān ... nivartate**] Cf. CS Śā 1.97ab; yas tv agnikalpān arthāñ jño jñātvā tebhyo nivartate T^{e}V^{e}G^{e}J2^{d}Ch^{d} **48 traya ... iti**] Cf. CS Sū 11.35; traya upastambhā iti — āhāraḥ, svapno, brahmacaryam iti T^{e}; traya upastambhā ity āhāraḥ svapno brahmacaryam iti V^{e}G^{e}(11.32) J2^{d}Ch^{d} **50 ebhis ... bhavati**] Cf. CS Sū 11.35; ebhis tribhir yuktiyuktair upastabdham upastambhaiḥ śarīraṃ ... T^{e}V^{e}G^{e}(11.32) J2^{d}Ch^{d} **51 śukraveganigrahaṇaṃ ṣāṇḍyakarāṇām**] CS Sū 25.40 śukraveganigrahaḥ ṣāṇḍyakarāṇāṃ T^{e}V^{e}G^{e}(25.39) J2^{d}Ch^{d}

48 traya ... brahmacaryam] Cf. AS Sū 9.18 tritayaṃ caitad upastambhanam āhāraḥ svapno 'brahmacaryaṃ ca. **50 ebhis ... bhavati**] Cf. AS Sū 9.18 ebhir yuktiyuktair upastabdham upastambhaiḥ śarīraṃ balavarṇopacayocitam anuvarttate yāvad āyuḥ saṃskāraḥ. **51 śukraveganigrahaṇaṃ ṣāṇḍyakarāṇām**] AS Sū 13.3 śukravegavinigrahaḥ ṣāṇḍhyakarāṇām

karāṇām. tathā, ***meḍhre vṛṣaṇayoś copadaṃśādi vyāpad bhavet pratihate tu śukra***. iti. tasmād yuktaṃ niṣevaṇam iti.

putrāyattā hi dharmādaya iti vyabhicāri, putravatām itareṣāṃ prāptidarśanāt. satyam etat. kintu vidhiparihāra< · · · >dharmādihānir na yathoktavidhyutpāditebhyaḥ satputrebhya iti.

putrasyāyatanaṃ vājīkaraṇam ity anekāntam, upayuktavājīkaraṇebhyo'pi stry utpatteḥ. atrāpi pūrva eva samādhiḥ.

athavā vājīkaraṇena śukravṛddhis tad vṛddhyā ca putrotpādaḥ. putraprādhānyāc caivam abhidhānam, duhitṛprāptāv api dharmādayo bhavanti. tathā hi smaraṇaṃ vaco,

---

54 prāptidarśanāt] (Ś^{e} p.840, *l*.1)prāptidarśanāt **56 iti ... 57 putrasyāyatanaṃ**] iti ⟨~~satputrebhya iti~~⟩(J^{d} p.18, *l*.1)putrasyāyatanaṃ **58 atrāpi**] atrā(M^{m} p.26, *l*.1)pi

---

śuklavega M^{m}J^{d}Ś^{e}; śutravegavi T^{d} ❀ **ṣāṇḍyakarāṇām**] Ś^{e}; ṣāṇḍyakaraṇan M^{m}; ṣāṇḍyakaraṇaṃ J^{d}; ṣaṇḍyakarāṇāṃ T^{d}
52 vṛṣaṇayoś copadaṃśādi] Ś^{e}; vṛṣaṇayoś cāpadaṃśādi M^{m}J^{d}; vṛṣaṇayo< · >di T^{d} **vyāpad**] J^{d}Ś^{e}; vyāpat M^{m}; yāvad T^{d} **53 śukra**] Ś^{e}; śukla M^{m}J^{d}; śutra T^{d} **54 putrāyattā**] M^{m}T^{d}Ś^{e}; putrāyattāḥ J^{d} ❀ **dharmādaya**] M^{m}T^{d}Ś^{e}; dharmādayaḥ J^{d} **55 vidhiparihāra<· · ·>dharmādi-**] M^{m}J^{d}; vidhipariha< · >dharmādi T^{d}; vidhiparihāra (dvārotpāditaputraiḥ) dharmādi Ś^{e} *em.* **56 -tebhyaḥ**] M^{m}J^{d}Ś^{e}; te⟨~~hi~~⟩bhyaḥ T^{d} **57 anekāntam**] M^{m}J^{d}Ś^{e}; anekāntā T^{d} ❀ **-bhyo 'pi**] J^{d}T^{d}Ś^{e}; bhyopi M^{m} **58 samādhiḥ**] M^{m}Ś^{e}; samādhi[-] J^{d}; sapimādhi< · > T^{d} **59 śukra-**] T^{d}Ś^{e}; śukla M^{m}J^{d} ❀ **putrotpādaḥ**] M^{m}J^{d}Ś^{e}; putrotpādaṃ T^{d} **61 smaraṇaṃ**] Ś^{e}; smārṇnaṃ M^{m}; smārnaṃ J^{d}T^{d}

---

52 tathā,] tathā J^{d}T^{d}Ś^{e} **53 śukra.**] śukla M^{m}J^{d}; śutra T^{d}; śukra Ś^{e} ❀ **iti.**[2]] J^{d}Ś^{e}; iti T^{d} **54 dharmādaya**] T^{d}Ś^{e}; dharmādayaḥ. J^{d} ❀ **vyabhicāri,**] Ś^{e}; vyabhicāri J^{d}T^{d} **56 iti.**] J^{d}Ś^{e}; iti T^{d} **57 anekāntam,**] M^{m}J^{d}Ś^{e}; anekāntā T^{d} **58 utpatteḥ.**] Ś^{e}; utpatter J^{d}T^{d} **samādhiḥ.**] Ś^{e}; samādhi[-] J^{d}; sapimādhi< · > T^{d} **59 putrotpādaḥ.**] J^{d}Ś^{e}; putrotpādaṃ T^{d} **60 abhidhānam,**] T^{d}; abhidhānaṃ J^{d}Ś^{e} ❀ **bhavanti.**] T^{d}Ś^{e}; bhavanti J^{d} **61 vaco,**] Ś^{e}; vaco J^{d}T^{d}

---

52 meḍhre ... 53 śukra] Cf. CS Sū 7.10; meḍhre vṛṣaṇayoḥ śūlam aṅgamardo hṛdi vyathā. bhavet pratihate śukre vibaddhaṃ mūtram eva ca. T^{e}V^{e}G^{e}Ch^{d}; meḍhre vṛṣāṇayoḥ śūle maṃgaṃdo hṛdi vyathā. bhavet pratihate śukre vibaṃdaṃ mūtram iva ca. J2^{d}

nāgnicin narakaṃ yāyāt na satputrī na kutracit.
<· · ·>janturyo 'dbhiḥ kanyāṃ prayacchati.

kiñca putrikāputrā apy abhyudayahetavaḥ. tathā hy aitihyam, *yayātiḥ kila svargāt paricyutaḥ putrikāputrair aṣṭakādibhiḥ svarga eva punaḥ prāpitaḥ.* iti. *evaṃ jaratkāror eva me putrāḥ putrikāputrāḥ.* iti. tasmād guṇavadapatyalābhād dharmādayaḥ, tasya ca putrasya hetur vājīkaraṇam iti, tad evaiṣṭavyam.

---

68 tad] (T^{d} p.25, *l.*1)tad

---

62 nāgnicin] M^{m}J^{d}Ś^{e}; <·>cin T^{d} ❁ **yāyāt]** Ś^{e}; yāyān M^{m}J^{d}; ya<·> T^{d} ❁ **kutracit 63 <· · ·>]** M^{m}; kutraci[-]<· · ·> J^{d}; kutra<·> T^{d}; kutracit. (satyavādī tathā) Ś^{e} *em.* **63 janturyo 'dbhiḥ]** Ś^{e}; janturyyodbhiḥ M^{m}; janturyodbhiḥ J^{d}; jantuyodbhiḥ T^{d} **64 abhyudaya-]** M^{m}T^{d}Ś^{e}; ubhaya T^{d} **65 paricyutaḥ]** M^{m}J^{d}Ś^{e}; paricyutaṃ T^{d} **66 jaratkāror eva]** M^{m}J^{d}Ś^{e}; ca vatkāro<·>va T^{d} **67 putrasya]** M^{m}J^{d}Ś^{e}; putrasya ca T^{d} **68 evaiṣṭavyam]** eveṣṭavyam M^{m}J^{d}T^{d}Ś^{e}

---

62 kutracit.] Ś^{e}; kutracit<· · ·> M^{m}; kutraci[-]<· · ·> J^{d}; kutra<·> T^{d} **64 -hetavaḥ.]** J^{d}Ś^{e}; hetavas T^{d} **66 prāpitaḥ.]** prāpita M^{m}J^{d}T^{d}Ś^{e} ❁ **iti.[1]]** J^{d}Ś^{e}; ity T^{d} **putrikāputrāḥ.]** putrikāputrā T^{d}Ś^{e}; putrikā[-]trā J^{d} **67 dharmādayaḥ,]** dharmādayaḥ Ś^{e}; dharmādayas J^{d}T^{d} **68 iti,]** iti J^{d}T^{d}Ś^{e}

---

62 nāgnicin … kutracit] Cf. Varāhapurāṇa 205.18ab; ŚKD 2.829 **63 <· · · >janturyo ... prayacchati]** The source is unidentified. **65 yayātiḥ … 66 prāpitaḥ]** Cf. Matsyapurāṇa 38-42 **66 evaṃ … putrikāputrāḥ]** The source is unidentified.

Translation*

lines 1–4 Since it has already been mentioned: **rejuvenation-therapy (*rasāyana*) is a sexual stimulant which brings about a healthy person's vitality** [CS Ci 1.1.5cd], then, rejuvenation-therapy may be [considered to be equivalent to] potency-therapy (*vājīkaraṇa*). However, it (i.e., potency-therapy) is not so in the present quarter. Therefore, [Ātreya] will explain the potency-therapy [and] its purpose [in this quarter]. Henceforth, then there is the commencement of [the chapter of] potency-therapy.

5–6 Likewise [as in the chapter of rejuvenation-therapy], a single chapter [of potency-therapy is divided] into four quarters (*pāda*). [Then,] it is said that the two [chapters, namely, CS Ci 1 and 2] are "paired chapters" (*adhyāya-dvaya*).

7–8 Since these [four quarters] beginning with this *Saṃyoga-śaramūlīya*-quarter form one chapter [of potency-therapy], everything beginning with the purpose of potency-therapy is mentioned in the *Saṃyoga-śaramūlīya*-quarter.

9–10 By the fact that the formula (*saṃyoga*) which consists of the roots of pen-reed grass (*śara-mūla*)[1] and so forth is found in this quarter, the very same quarter in the chapter of potency-therapy is [called] *Saṃyoga-śaramūlīya*-quarter.

---

* At the beginning of this quarter, Ś^{e} and the other editions and manuscripts of CS put the opening phrase: "Now, we shall explain the quarter in the chapter of potency-therapy, [called] *Saṃyoga-śaramūlīya*[-quarter]. Thus, indeed spoke the lord Ātreya." However, all of the copies of the manuscript of Jajjaṭa's *Nirantarapadavyākhyā* omit this opening phrase.

[1] *Śara*: pen-reed grass; *Saccharum sara* Roxb. or *Saccharum bengalense* Retz.

11–12 **A self-disciplined man should always seek potency-therapy (*vājīkaraṇa*) afterward** [CS Ci 2.1.3ab]. Thus beginning, the potency-therapy is indeed that by which [a man] is made [to be] like a horse, like a stallion.

13–14 [The author says:] ***By which (i.e., potency-therapy), being very strong like a stallion, he goes to women [for making love] without interruption*** [CS Ci 1.1.9cd]. So it is, [yet some may ask:] that why does not occur the loss of primary tissue (i.e., semen) of him whose tissues are [already] accumulated on account of the rejuvenation-therapy?[2]

15–16 The word *anu* [in *anv icchet*] is appropriate for many meanings ⟨. . .⟩, [but in this case], the meaning 'afterwards' is what is used, namely, 'after lovemaking'.

17–19 The word 'man' (*puruṣa*) excludes boys and very old men. [The author] will say: ***Since, when a very young boy, whose every tissue is undeveloped, has sexual intercourse with women, he [at once would be scorched] like a waterless pond*** [CS Ci 2.4.41].

20–21 ***Likewise, if an old man makes love to a woman, he would instantly fall to pieces like a dry, rough, insect-eaten, decrepit piece of wood when he is touched*** [CS Ci 2.4.42].

22 Moreover, there is no need to [say that the word 'man'] excludes women and eunuchs, because potency-therapy is not applicable to them.

23–25 The word 'always' (*nitya*) is known to mean 'constantly' or 'the act of frequenting'. Rejuvenation-therapy, when it is applied in this way, fattens all of the tissues. [However,] this is not the case with potency-therapy, because it (i.e., potency-therapy),

[2] The answer is given in lines 24–25.

when it is constantly used just like eating of food, upholds the growth of [only] one tissue, semen, thus [it is said].

26–29 By the word 'self-disciplined' (*ātmavat*), [the author] effects 'resolution', hence, 'command'. The man, who is able to restrain himself from other men's wives, etc., by his resolution, is referred to [here]. He does not have illicit intercourse with a woman, just like an animal [does, thus] transgressing [the command] ⟨...⟩. At all times, [the following] is mentioned for the sake of the necessity of reference to him whose senses are restrained.

30–31 **When [he acquires] duty (*dharma*) and prosperity (*artha*); likewise, fondness (*prīti*) and surely fame (*yaśas*)** [CS Ci 2.1.3cd], **this [potency-therapy] would become a place for the son; and these qualities (i.e., duty, prosperity, fondness and fame) would also be seats of the son** [CS Ci 2.1.4ab].

32–33 Thus, it is said that duty, prosperity, fondness and fame are necessary to have a son. How is it said that those beginning with duty, are seats of the son? [This is because] duty [etc.] are [necessary] for begetting of the son. And also, the revealed tradition (*śruti*) says:

34–35 *[When he is born,] the brahmin becomes a debtor by means of [these] three debts, [namely,] the Agnihotṛ-sacrifice belongs to the gods, the celibacy (*brahmacarya*) belongs to the seers, [and] progeny belongs to the ancestors. Thus, the world is not without a son.*

36 [Moreover,] *indeed [like] all animals, those who know [this* śruti*] never carry out union with [their] mother.*

37–38 Or again, ⟨...⟩ [a son] causes the parents to do their duty, and when he has acquired wealth even from another, he offers [it to the parents]. And fondness and pride [are felt by the parents] from looking at [their] son. And the venerable Vyāsa says:

39 *Of pleasure and pain, there is no[thing] better than the generation of a son [and nothing worse than] the separation [of the son].*

40–41 And he (i.e., the son) extends the fondness of the parents on account of being a virtuous son. [Hence,] these qualities (i.e., duty, prosperity, fondness and fame) would be the seats of the son. Therefore, the statement: **[A self-disciplined man] should [always] seek potency-therapy afterward (*vājīkaraṇam anv icchet*)** [CS Ci 2.1.3ab] is reasonable.

42–43 On the occasion of renouncing the world, it is said that he should take recourse in the duty which is promoting and characterised by the attainment of heaven. The instruction says:

44 **As a silkworm gathers up threads which bring about its death** [CS Śā 1.96ab], **[so an ignorant man (*ajña*) acts in the same way].**

45 **[However,] an intelligent man (*jña*), after knowing that some sense objects have a fire-like quality, keeps away from them** [CS Śā 1.97ab]. **[Because of his lack of initiation [and] lack of contact, he does not expose himself to that misfortune.]**[3]

46–47 The instruction of celibacy (*brahmacarya*) takes recourse to the duty (*dharma*) leading to final bliss

---

[3]Jajjaṭa quotes only CS Śā 1.96ab and 97ab, and omits CS Śā 1.96cd and 97cd here.

CS Śā 1.96ab: *koṣakāro yathā hy aṃśūn upādatte vadhapradān.*

CS Śā 1.96cd: *upārasāyanadatte tathārthebhyas tṛṣṇām ajñaḥrasāyana sadāturaḥ.*

CS Śā 1.97ab: *yas tv agnikalpān arthāñ jño jñātvā tebhyo nivartate.*

CS Śā 1.97cd: *anārambhād asaṃyogāt taṃ duḥkhaṃ nopatiṣṭhate.*

(*naiḥśreyasika*), and it is said that this [instruction of celibacy] brings a good result (*abhyudaya*), [therefore] there is no disagreement arising from the mutual contradiction [between celibacy and potency-therapy]. So should it be, [and it is instructed:]

48–49 ***There are three supports, namely, food, sleep, and celibacy. By these three [supports], [the human body is] maintained*** [CS Sū 11.35], and so forth. [Then,] why is "frequent visiting of women" (*strī-niṣevaṇa*) [CS Ci 1.1.9cd paraphrased][4] mentioned in this context?

50 [The answer is that] since [it says]: ***The body is maintained by these three [supports when the three supports are] under proper conditions* (yukti-yuktaiḥ*)*** [CS Sū 11.35].

51–53 And in case of the retention of semen, [such a condition] would be regarded as "a defilement" (or "morbid condition") (*doṣa*), [and it is said]: ***Among the causes of impotency, the suppression of semen's flow* (śukra-vega-nigrahaṇa*) [is the most serious]*** [CS Sū 25.40], and likewise, [it is said]: ***When semen is impeded, there would be disorder[s] beginning with a kind of venereal disease* (upadaṃśa*) in the penis and of the testicles*** [CS Sū 7.10]. Therefore, it is said that "frequent visiting [of women]" (*[strī]niṣevaṇa*) is appropriate.

54–56 [The statement]: "[These qualities] beginning with duty depend on a son" (*putrāyattā hi dharmādayaḥ*) [CS Ci 2.1.4ab paraphrased] may be debatable for other ones than those who have [virtuous] sons. This is true. However, [some say] that ⟨...⟩ [because of sons begotten by means of] avoiding the

[4] See the lines 13–14.

precepts, there is breach of the law, not because of virtuous sons who have been begotten according to the previously mentioned precepts.

57–58 [The statement]: "potency-therapy would become a place for the son" (*putrasyāyatanaṃ vājīkaraṇam*) [CS Ci 2.1.4a paraphrased] is uncertain, because there is also the production of a female from the proper use of potency-therapy. Also in this case, it is previously approved.

59–61 Or, the increase of semen is by means of potency-therapy, and the production of a son is by means of its (i.e., semen's) increase. And because of the supremacy of son, the word 'son' (*putra*) is thus [used], [but] even in the acquisition of a daughter, there occur those beginning with duty. For thus, there are traditionally sanctioned words:

62 *[The one] who arranges [the sacrificial] fire should not go to hell; [the one who has] the virtuous daughter should not go anywhere.*

63 *⟨...⟩ [Thus, a truth-speaking] man is [one] who gives a young girl in marriage along with water.*

64 [Furthermore,] a daughter's sons, who by agreement become the sons of [her] father (*putrikā-putra*),[5] are also the causes of happiness. For thus, the tradition has said:

65–66 *Yayāti (king of the lunar race), they say, fallen from heaven, attained the same heaven again by means of his daughters' sons who by agreement become [Yayāti['']s] sons (*putrikā-putra*), beginning with Aṣṭaka.*

Thus, just like Jaratkāru['']s [sons], my sons are my daughters' sons who by agreement become [my] sons

[5]For *putrikā*, see MDh 9.127; *Bṛhaspatismṛti* 1.26.82; BauDhS 2.2.3.15, 31, 32.

(putrikā-putra).

67–68 Therefore, it should certainly be accepted that from the acquisition of offspring (*apatya*) possessing good qualities, there are those beginning with duty; and that the reason for the [birth of] a son is potency-therapy. [Therefore] this (i.e., potency-therapy) is indeed to be desired.

Further reading

Ācārya, Yādavaśarman Trivikrama (ed.) 1941. *Maharṣiṇā Punarvasunopadiṣṭā, tacchiṣyeṇāgniveśena praṇītā, Caraka-Dṛḍhabalābhyāṃ pratisaṃskṛtā Carakasaṃhitā, śrīCakrapāṇidattaviracitayā āyurvedadīpikāvyākhyayā saṃvalitā*. Mumbayyāṃ: Nirṇayasāgara Mudrāyantrālaye, 3rd edn.

Āgāśe, Kāśīnāthaśāstrī and Narahariśāstri Taḷekara (eds.) 1959–1978. *Kṛṣṇayajurvedīyataittirīyasaṃhitā, ŚrīmatSāyaṇācāryaviracitabhāṣyasametā*, vol. 42 of *Ānandāśrama Sanskrit Series*. Pune: Gaṅgādhara Bāpūrāva Kāḷe.

Āṭhavale, Anaṃta Dāmodara (ed.) 1980. *Aṣṭāṅgasaṅgrahaḥ. ŚrīmadVṛddhavāgbhaṭaviracitaḥ Induvyākhyāsahitaḥ*. Puṇe: Maheśa Anaṃta Āṭhavale, Śrīmad Ātreya Prakāśanam.

Bhaṭṭācāryya, Jīvānanda Vidyāsāgara (ed.) 1876. *Dharmaśāstrasaṅgrahaḥ = Dharmashastra Sangraha, or Atri, Vishnu, Harita, Yajnavalka [sic], Ushana, Angira, Yama, Apastamba, Samvartha [sic], Katyayana, Vrihaspati, Parasara, Vyasa, Shankha, Likhita, Daksha, Goutama, Shatatapa, and Vashistha [sic]*. Kalikātā: Sarasvatīyantrayantra. 2 parts in one volume.

— 1877. *Caraka-saṃhitā ... SrīJīvānandaVidyāsāgara-Bhaṭṭācāryeṇa ... saṃskṛtā ... = Charak sanhitā, or, Digest of Charaka. The most Ancient and Authoritative System of Hindu Medicine Taught by Punarvashu and Written by his Disciple Agnibesha, modified and arranged by Charaka in Eight Divisions – Sūtra,*

Nidāna, Vimāna, Sharīra, Indria, Chikitsita, Kalpa and Siddhi. Calcutta: The editor, 1st edn. Printed at the Saraswatī Press, Calcutta by Kshetramohan Mukerji.

Gaṅgāviṣṇu Śrīkṛṣṇadāsa (ed.) 1932. *Śrīmanmaharṣipravaracarakapraṇītā Carakasaṃhitā, āyurvedoddhārakavaidyapañcānanavaidyaratnarājavaidyapaṇḍitarāmaprasādavaidyopādhyāyaviracitā evaṃ āyurvedācārya paṃ. Śivaśarmaṇā saṃśodhitā prasādanībhāṣāṭīkāsahitā.* Bambaī: Lakṣmīveṅkaṭeśvara Steam Press.

Haridatta Śāstrin (ed.) 1941. *Maharṣipunarvasuśiṣyeṇa ṛṣivareṇa agniveśena praṇītā mahāmuninā carakeṇa kāpilabalena dṛḍhabalena ca pratisaṃkṛtā Carakasaṃhitā mahāmahopādhyāyacarakacaturānanaśrīcakrapāṇidattaviracitayā Āyurvedadīpikāvyākhyayā (tathā cikitsāsthānataḥ siddhisthānaṃ yāvat) śrīvāgabhaṭaśiṣyācāryavarajajjaṭaviracitayā Nirantarapadavyākhyayā ca saṃvalitā | Āyurvedācāryeṇa Paṇ. Śrīharidattaśāstriṇā saṃśodhitā, pūritajajjaṭaṭīkātruṭitāṃśabhāgā ca.* Lahore: Motilal Banarsidass, 2nd edn.

Kuṃṭe, Ananta Moreśvara, Kṛṣṇaśāstrī Rāma candra Navare, and Hariśāstrī Parādkar (eds.) 1902. *Aṣṭāṅgahṛdayam, śrīmadVāgbhaṭaviracitam, sūtra-śārīra-nidāna-cikitsā-kalpa-uttarasthānavibhaktam śrīmadAruṇadattapraṇītayā sarvāṃgasuṃdaryākhyayā vyākhyayā samalaṃkṛtam,* vol. 3 of *Kṛṣṇadāsa Āyurveda Sīrīja.* Muṃbayyām: Nirṇayasāgara Press.

Kuṃṭe, Ananta Moreśvara and Kṛṣṇaśāstrī Rāmacandra Navare (eds.) 1982. *Aṣṭāṅgahṛdayam, śrīmadvāgbhaṭaviracitam, sūtra-śārīra-nidāna-cikitsā-kalpa-uttarasthānavibhaktam śrīmadaruṇadattapraṇītayā sarvāṃgasuṃdaryākhyayā vyākhyayā samalaṃkṛtam,* vol. 4 of *Kṛṣṇadāsa Āyurveda Sīrīja.* Varanasi and Delhi: Chaukhambha Orientalia, 7th edn.

Kunjan Pillai, Suranad 1957. *Alphabetical index of the Sanskrit manuscripts in the University Manuscripts Library,*

Trivandrum. Trivandrum: Suranad Kunjan Pillai. From v. 3 entitled: *Alphabetical index ... in the Oriental Research Institute and Manuscripts Library, Trivandrum*.

Nene, Gopāla Śāstrī (ed.) 1970. *Manusmṛtiḥ. Kullūkabhaṭṭapraṇīta 'Manvarthamuktāvalī' ṭīkāsahita-'Maṇiprabhā' hindīvyākhyopetā, kṣepakapariśiṣṭaślokaiḥ, ślokānukramaṇikayā ca sahitā. Hindīvyākhyākāraḥ Haragovindaśāstrī. Sampādakaḥ Gopālaśāstrī Nene*, vol. 114 of *Haridāsasaṃskṛtagranthamālāsamākhya Kāśīsaṃskṛtasīrizpustakamālā*. Banārasa Siṭī: Caukhambā Saṃskṛta Sīriz Āphisa.

Rādhākānta, Rājā 1876. *Shabda kalpadrumah, or, The tree bearing all the words that may be wished for*. Calcutta: New Bengal Press.

Śāstrin, K. Mahādeva 1939. *A Descriptive Catalogue of Sanskrit Manuscripts in the Curator's Office Library*. Trivandrum: V. V. Press Branch.

Weber, Albrecht 1964. *Śrīśuklayajurvede Śatapathabrāhmaṇam...Mādhyandīyāṃ śākhām anusṛtya śrīmatsāyaṇācāryaharisvāmīdvivedagaṅgakṛtabhāṣyebhyaḥ sāram uddhṛtya*, vol. 96 of *Caukhambā-Saṃskṛta-granthamālā*. Vāraṇāsī: Caukhāṃbā Saṃskṛta Sīrīja āphīsa, 2nd edn. Contains the text of the Brāhmaṇa and extracts from the commentaries of Sayana, Harisvāmin and Dvivedagaṅga.

Zysk, Kenneth G. 2009. "Sanskrit Commentaries on the Carakasaṃhitā with Special Reference to Jajjaṭa's Nirantarapadavyākhyā." *eJournal of Indian Medicine*, **2**, 83–99.

9

P. Ram Manohar

Glimpses of the *Siddhamantra*

Introduction

The *Siddhamantra* is a short treatise on pharmacology in Ayurveda that was composed by Keśava, a renowned physician scholar who lived in the 13th century CE.[1] This work is historically important for theoretical innovations that have been put forth by the author to explain drug action with greater clarity and precision. The treatise is very short, (*atyalpam*, in the words of the author himself) leaving ample scope for discussions and interpretations. But for the elaborate commentary *Prakāśa* composed by Vopadeva, the son of the author, much of the thought process involved in construction of the new theories would have perhaps remained in oblivion.

[1]"Thus, the date of Keśava is fixed as the first half of the 13th Cent. AD" (Sharma 1977: 2, intro. p. 4), and "since Keśava appears to have been the royal physician of Siṃharāja, who is usually identified with Siṃhaṇa or Singhaṇa II, one of the Yādava kings of Devagiri, who reigned from A.D. 1210 to A.D. 1247, he lived during the first half of the thirteenth century" (Meulenbeld 1999–2002: IIA, 186).

Publications of *Siddhamantra*

The book was published first in 1898 without the commentary and later in 1977 by Priya Vrat Sharma with the commentary in Sanskrit.[2] Priya Vrat Sharma had access to five manuscripts of the text apart from the 1898 printed edition, but there is still room for a meticulous critical edition of the work today. The British Library in London reportedly has a copy of the 1898 edition of *Siddhamantraprakāśa*.[3] Meulenbeld gives a brief description of Keśava in his monumental work *History of Indian Medical Literature*. In the bibliography, he lists two other editions of *Siddhamantra* edited by Morarji Vaidya and Yadavji Trikamji Acharya in 1908 and 1975 respectively.[4]

Sharma and Meulenbeld have discussed in fairly great detail about the author, the date of the text, the comment-

---

[2]Pade and Bhālacandra 1898, Sharma 1977.

[3]Priya Vrat Sharma states in his introduction, "It was published in 1898 at the Jñānasāgara Press, duly edited by Vaidya Śaṅkaradāji Śāstrī Pade with the assistance of Śrī Bhālacandra. This publication is entitled *Siddhamantraprakāśa* though there is no commentary. In fact, the text is *Siddhamantra* and the commentary is known as *Prakāśa*. In introduction, the editor has remarked that the work was not available at that time (as now)" (Sharma 1977: section 2, intro. p. 3).

[4]Meulenbeld lists additional printed editions of *Siddhamantra* not mentioned by P. V. Sharma: "**a** ed., together with another work called *Yogeśvara*, under the common title of *Āyurvedasaṃgraha*, by Vaidya Śaṃkara Dājī Śāstrī Pade, with the assistance of Śrī Bhālacandra, Jñānasāgara Press, Bombay 1898 ...; the title of this publication is *Siddhamantra Prakāśa*, though the commentary is absent (P. V. Sharma's Introduction to the *Siddhamantra*. 3); ... ***b** ed. by Morarji Vaidya of Bombay, 1908/09 ..., ***c** ed. by Vaidya Yadavji Trikamji Acharya (together with the *vātaghnatvādinirṇaya* of Nārāyaṇa Bhiṣaj ..., **d** Vopadeva's *Hṛdayadīpaka Nighaṇṭu* and *Siddhamantra* of Vaidyācārya Keśava with *Prakāśa* Commentary of Vopadeva, ed. by Priya Vrat Sharma, Chaukhamba Ayurveda Granthamala 1, Amarabharati Prakashan, Varanasi, 1977." (Meulenbeld 1999–2002: IIA, 212–13).

ary, the historical context as well as the contents of the text and the commentary in his introduction. This does not, however, rule out the scope for a fresh enquiry into the work. In fact, *Siddhamantra* deserves more serious attention from the students and practitioners of Ayurveda than has been meted out to it. A comprehensive translation is very much desirable and the text should also be approached with a critical and analytical bent of mind.

The subject matter of *Siddhamantra*

Siddhamantra can be approximately translated as "the infallible or fail-safe hymn" and the title promises immediate and surefire practical results to those who access the work. In this context, the word *siddha* can be interpreted as "tested and proven effective".[5] In other words, this treatise is claimed to be as effective as a tested mantra or hymn. Suśruta has also referred to tested and effective formulations as a potent mantra.[6] In one context he states that the formulations that have been vouchsafed by authorities and which produce tangible results can be used like a mantra without the need for logical analysis. Vāgbhaṭa compares a tested medicine with a potent mantra.[7] The author claims that the work is composed to enable the physicians to comprehend the principle (*tattva*) of drug potency (*dravyaśakti*)

---

[5]The *Vācaspatyam* encyclopedia considers the word *siddha* to indicate "rock salt, king, maturity, sage, divine being," etc. (Bhaṭṭācārya 1969–1970: 5293). Monier-Williams' dictionary interprets *siddha* as "accomplished, successful, perfected, sacred, illustrious," etc. (Monier-Williams *et al.* 1899: 1215).

[6]*Suśrutasaṃhitā*, cikitsāsthāna 1, 76ab (Ācārya 1938: 403): *mantravat saṃprayoktavyo na mīmāṃsyaḥ kathañ cana*|

[7]*Aṣṭāṅgahṛdayasaṃhitā*, uttarasthāna 40, 81 (Kuṃṭe *et al.* 1902: 954): *idam āgamasiddhatvāt pratyakṣaphaladarśanāt mantravat saṃprayoktavyaṃ na mīmāṃsyaṃ kathañ cana 81*|

quickly (*drāk*) and easily (*sukhena*).[8] A physician who is well versed with the knowledge of potency and action of drugs can indeed become successful in clinical practice. Drug potency means ability of the drug to alleviate disease. Like a fail-safe *mantra*, it can be applied with ease and reaps rich dividends. In other words, it is as short and powerful as a *mantra*.

The opening verse invokes Dhanvantari and is a eulogy in praise of his contributions towards revealing the properties of medicinal plants. This appears to be an allusion to the *Dhanvantarinighaṇṭu*, which must have enjoyed a high reputation in the time of the author.[9] This invocation has a double meaning.[10] The salient features of the *Siddhamantra* can be summarized as follows:

1. Reverse approach to pharmacological evaluation of drugs.
2. Classification of drugs into 48 (57) subgroups under eight broad groups based on reverse pharmacological attributes.
3. Reconciliation of contradictions in the views of authorities in the field of Ayurveda.
4. Construction of theories to facilitate reconciliation of contradictions.
5. Achieving brevity in effectively compressing a vast subject into the space of less than a couple of hundred verses.

---

[8]Keśava summarizes the purpose of composing his work thus (Sharma 1977: section 2, p. 2): *granthaḥ saṃgranthyate 'ty alpaṃ siddhamantrāhvayo mayā, vaidyāḥ sukhena drāk dravyaśaktitattvam vitantv iti|*

[9]Meulenbeld dates the *Dhanvantarinighaṇṭu* to the eleventh century (1999–2002: IIA, 173).

[10]The invocation with which the *Siddhamantra* begins is (Sharma 1977: section 2, p. 2): *āyurvedasudhāṃbodhisārasāraṇikā giraḥ| ullāsitauṣadhagrāmaḥ jayanty amṛtajanmanaḥ|*

I shall now review these features in greater detail.

The reverse approach to pharmacology

The uniqueness of *Siddhamantra* is the reverse approach to pharmacology adopted by the author. Deviating from the tradition of elaborating the taste (*rasa*), properties (*guṇa*), potency (*vīrya*), post-digestive state (*vipāka*) empirically observed activity (*prabhāva*) and then inferring the action on humours (*doṣa*),[11] *Siddhamantra* enlists substances in 57 categories depending on their action on the humours (*doṣa*). The original contribution of *Siddhamantra* lies not in simply listing the action of substances on the humours (*doṣa*), but the precision with which the action is delineated.[12]

The knowledge of taste (*rasa*) and other pharmacological principles of a drug do not constitute an end in itself. They are the means to understand the activity of the drug or food substance in terms of the effect on the humours (*doṣa*). Available works on Ayurveda discuss in greater detail about taste (*rasa*), properties (*guṇa*), potency (*vīrya*), and post-digestive state (*vipāka*) and are less explicit when it comes to the net effect they have on the balance of the humours. Things are further complicated by the fact that differences in opinion are also seen amongst the authorities in the field and it becomes quite a task for the average

[11]Meulenbeld (2001), "Reflections on the Basic Concepts of Indian Pharmacology," provides an excellent review of the classical approach to understanding drug action in the tradition of Ayurveda.

[12]Keśava explains that the taste (*rasa*), properties (*guṇa*), potency (*vīrya*), and post-digestive state (*vipāka*) of a drug constitute the means to determine the action of the drug on the humours (*doṣa*). His work, he says, deals with the effect of substances on the humours (*doṣa*), which is the end itself and so he does not discuss the therapeutic means, i.e., *rasa, guṇa, vīrya* and *vipāka* (Sharma 1977: section 2, p. 2): *rasavīryavipākair hi dravyaśaktir vivicyate| kope śame vā doṣāṇāṃ sātra spaṣṭā na tena te|*

physician to make proper decisions in the clinic. The *Siddhamantra* is an attempt to fill this gap.

Classification of substances into 48 (57) subgroups under eight broad groups

The *Siddhamantra* is a strikingly terse piece of literary work and there are just nine verses in the text that sum up the conceptual basis on which drugs and food articles are classified into 57 categories indicating their impact on the humours (*doṣa*). According to Vopadeva, the commentator, these nine verses are together known in Sanskrit as the *navaślokī*.[13] The enumeration of these substances in these 57 categories is achieved in the remaining 160 verses making a total of 169 verses. The classification of substances enlisted in the *Siddhamantra* is structured and logical. The text considers in a precise manner how a given herb or food substance can affect the humour (*doṣa*) by either pacifying it or disturbing it. These effects are computed for all the logical possible combinations and permutations of the three humours (*doṣa*) forming eight broad groups in all: wind (*vāta*), bile (*pitta*), phlegm (*kapha*), wind-bile (*vātapitta*), wind-phlegm (*vātakapha*), phlegm-bile (*kaphapitta*), pacifying the three humours (*tridoṣahara*) and disturbing the three humours (*tridoṣakara*). The eight broad categories become fifteen when we consider the pacifying and aggravating effect on the *doṣas*. They further expand into fifty-seven specific subgroups indicative of the varied im-

[13]Vopadeva states at the end of his commentary on the ninth verse of the *Siddhamantra* that the section of nine verses, or *navaślokī*, concludes here (Sharma 1977: section 2, p. 12): *iti vopadevīyasiddhamantraprakāśe navaślokī*|

pact on the humours (*doṣa*).[14] The expanded list according to Vopadeva is as follows:

I. *vātaghna* group (the *vāta* pacifiers)

1 *vātaghna*
Pacifies *vāta* in isolation as well as *vāta* associated with *pitta* and *kapha* separately or together but it neither pacifies nor aggravates *pitta* and *kapha* in isolation; the same logic applies in all the 'pacifying (*-ghna*)' subgroups[15]

2 *vātapittaghna*

3 *vātaśleṣmaghna*

4 *vātaghnapittala*
Pacifies *vāta* in isolation as well as *vāta* associated with *kapha*, but it aggravates *vāta* associated with *pitta* as well as *pitta* in isolation, same logic applies in all the 'aggravating (*-la*)' subgroups[16]

5 *vātaghnaśleṣmala*

6 *vātaghnapittaśleṣmala*

7 *vātaghnapittodāsīna*
Pacifies *vāta* only in isolation, does not aggravate or pacify *vāta* associated with *pitta* and *kapha* or *pitta* and *kapha* in isolation, same logic applies in all the 'neutral (*-udāsīna*)' subgroups[17]

---

[14] Keśava summarizes the classification system of drugs based on their action on the *doṣas* (*ibid.*): *vāte pitte kaphe vātapitte vātakaphe kramāt, kaphapitte triṣu hitavargāḥ saptahito 'ṣṭamaḥ|*

[15] Illustrative definition of a *vātaghna* drug (Sharma 1977: section 2, p. 11): *vātaghnam eva yad dravyaṃ tad vātam hanti kevalam| sānyaṃ ca kevalāvanyau na hanti na karoti ca|*

[16] Illustrative definition of a *vātaghna* drug that aggravates other *doṣas* (*ibid.*): *vātaghnam anyajananaṃ dravyaṃ yad hanti tac calam| kevalaṃ kevalau sānyāv anyo vardhayate malau|*

[17] Illustrative definition of a *vātaghna* drug that is neutral on other *doṣas* (*ibid.*): *vātaghnam anyodāsīnaṃ yat tac chuddhānilāpahaṃ| śuddhau sānyau na hanty anyau na karotīti sarvataḥ|*

8 *vātaghnaśleṣmodasina*
9 *vātaghnapittaśleṣmodasina*

II. *pittaghna* group (the *pitta* pacifiers)

1 *aghna*
2 *pittaśleṣmaghna*
3 *pittavātaghna*
4 *pittaghnavātala*
5 *pittaghnaśleṣmala*
6 *pittaghnavātaśleṣmala*
7 *pittaghnavātodāsīna*
8 *pittaghnaśleṣmodāsīna*
9 *pittaghnavātaśleṣmodāsīna*

III. *śleṣmaghna* group (the *śleṣma* pacifiers)

1 *śleṣmaghna*
2 *śleṣmavātaghna*
3 *śleṣmapittaghna*
4 *śleṣmaghnavātala*
5 *śleṣmaghnapittala*
6 *śleṣmaghnavātapittala*
7 *śleṣmaghnavātodāsīna*
8 *śleṣmaghnapittodāsīna*
9 *śleṣmaghnavātapittodāsīna*

IV. *vātapittaghna* group (the *vātapitta* pacifiers)

1 *vātapittaghna*
2 *vātapittaghnaśleṣmala*
3 *vātapittaghnaśleṣmodāsīna*

V. *vātaśleṣmaghna* group (the *vātaśleṣma* pacifiers)

1 *vātaśleṣmaghna*
2 *vātaśleṣmaghnapittala*
3 *vātaśleṣmaghnapittodāsīna*

VI. *pittaśleṣmaghna* group (the *pittaśleṣma* pacifiers)

1 *pittaśleṣmaghna*
2 *pittaśleṣmaghnavātala*

3 *pittaśleṣmaghnavātodāsīna*

VII. *doṣaghna* group (the *tridoṣa* pacifiers)

1 *vātapittaśleṣmaghna*

VIII. *doṣodāsīna* group (the *tridoṣa* neutrals)

1 *vātapittaśleṣmodāsīna*

IX. *vātala* group (the *vāta* aggravators)

1 *vātala*
2 *vātalapittodāsīna*
3 *vātalaśleṣmodāsīna*
4 *vātalapittaśleṣmodāsīna*

X. *pittala* group (the *pitta* aggravators)

1 *pittala*
2 *pittalavātodāsīna*
3 *pittalaśleṣmodāsīna*
4 *pittalavātaśleṣmodāsīna*

XI. *śleṣmala* group (the *śleṣma* aggravators)

1 *śleṣmala*
2 *śleṣmalapittodāsīna*
3 *śleṣmalavātodāsīna*
4 *śleṣmalavātapittodāsīna*

XII. *vātapittala* group (the *vātapitta* aggravators)

1 *vātapittala*
2 *vātapittalaśleṣmodāsīna*

XIII. *pittaśleṣmala* group (the *pittaśleṣma* aggravators)

1 *pittaśleṣmala*
2 *pittaśleṣmalavātodāsīna*

XIV. *vātaśleṣmala* group (the *vātaśleṣma* aggravators)

1 *vātaśleṣmala*
2 *vātaśleṣmalapittodāsīna*

XV. *doṣala* group (the *tridoṣa* aggravators)

1 *vātapittaśleṣmala*

In this classification, it appears as though the *vātapittaghna* and *vātaśleṣmaghna* subgroups under the *vātaghna* group (I.)

and the *pittaśleṣmaghna* subgroup under the *pittaghna* group (II.) are repeated in the *vātapittaghna*, *vātaśleṣmaghna* and *pittaśleṣmaghna* groups mentioned later (IV, V, and VI respectively). Vopadeva clarifies that in the case of the subgroup *vātapittaghna* falling under the *vātaghna* group, *vāta* is dominant and *pitta* has only a secondary association, whereas in the *vātapittaghna*, both *vāta* and *pitta* are equally dominant.[18]

Both Vopadeva and Sharma have encountered difficulties in listing the 57 groups that can be derived based on the action of substances on the humours (*doṣa*). In fact, Keśava does not give the number 57 and only mentions eight broad categories that can be sub-classified further. Vopadeva in his commentary gives the detailed list, which has been tabulated by Sharma. Vopadeva says that there are nine subgroups under the *vātaghna* group, but he actually lists only seven of them, i.e.,

1. *vātaghna*,
2. *vātaghnapittala*,
3. *vātaghnaśleṣmala*,
4. *vātaghnapittaśleṣmala*,
5. *vātaghnapittodāsīna*,
6. *vātaghnaśleṣmodāsīna*,
7. *vātaghnapittaśleṣmodāsīna*.

Sharma lists eight subgroups under *vātaghna* by adding *vātapittaghna* and *vātaśleṣmaghna* but omitting *vātaghnapittaśleṣmodāsīna* mentioned by Vopadeva. Sharma, however, lists nine subgroups under *pittaghna* and *śleṣmaghna* groups by adding *pittaśleṣmaghna*, *pittavātaghna* and *śleṣmavātaghna*, *śleṣmapittaghna* subgroups respectively. In addition, *vātaśleṣmaghna* and *pittaśleṣmaghna* groups are listed separately.

[18]Vopadeva clarifies that there is no overlap in the subgroups: *sapitte vāte vātaprādhānyam vāte pitte tūbhayaprādhānyam vācyam ity asaṅkaraḥ|*

This leads to repetition of these categories as subgroups under *vātaghna* and *pittaghna* groups as well as independent groups.

Vopadeva mentions that variant groups like *vātaghnapittalālpakapha* can also be derived from this classification as this becomes necessary when fixing the properties of a drug in a very precise manner.[19]

In fact, it is not sure whether Keśava ever attempted to fit the substances listed in his work under 57 categories. The actual categories under which Keśava lists medicinal and food substances are quite different from the mathematical subgroups given by Vopadeva and Sharma. Keśava categorizes substances on the basis of actually-observed properties (*yatra dravye yo dṛṣṭaḥ sa tatrokta eva*). Keśava's listing is given below and makes 48 subgroups under eight major groups.

I. *vātaghna varga*
   1. *vātaghna*, e.g., *Modakī*,
   2. *vātaghnaśleṣmala*, e.g., *Asthiśṛṅkhalā*,
   3. *vātaghnapittakaphakṛt*, e.g., *Miśreyā*,
   4. *vātaghnapittalālpakapha*, e.g., *Ākṣikīsurā*,
   5. *vātaghnapittakarakapha*, e.g., *Tilataila*,
   6. *vātaghnalpapittaśleṣma*, e.g., *Madhumāraka*,
   7. *vātaghnapittakaphodāsīna*, e.g., *Masūrayūṣa*,
   8. *vātaghnaśleṣmalapittodāsīna*, e.g., *Palāndu*

II. *pittaghna varga*
   1. *pittaghna*, e.g., *Candana*,
   2. *pittaghnavātakara*, e.g., *Sipi (gundrā)*,
   3. *pittaghnaśleṣmala*, e.g., *Śālmalī*,

---

[19]Vopadeva explains that further variants are possible but can be resolved into the main groups to avoid infinite regress (Sharma 1977: section 2, p. 12): *vātaghnapittalālpaśleṣmalādayas taratamabhedā vātaghnapittalaśleṣmalādyantarbhūtatvād anantatvāc ca na gaṇitāḥ|*

4. *pittaghnavātakaphakṛt*, e.g., *Marsaśāka*,
5. *pittaghnavātakaphodāsīna*, e.g., *Phalgu*,
6. *pittaghnakaphodāsīna*, e.g., *Bimbī*

III. *kaphaghna varga*
1. *kaphaghna*, e.g., *Sāla*,
2. *kaphaghnavātala*, e.g., *Rakta Śigru* (flower and shoot),
3. *kaphaghnapittala*, e.g., *Brahmasomā*,
4. *kaphaghnapittavātakṛt*, e.g., *Droṇapuṣpī*,
5. *kaphaghnavātalapittodāsīna*, e.g., *Veṇupatrī*,
6. *kaphaghnapittalavatodāsīna*, e.g., *Madhu (Auddālaka)*,
7. *kaphaghnapittavatodāsīna*, e.g., *Drakṣāsava*,
8. *kaphaghnavātakṛtpittodāsīna*, e.g., *Kharjūramadya*

IV. *vātapittaghna varga*
1. *vātapittahara*, e.g., *Śākavṛkṣa*,
2. *vātapittaghnaśleṣmala*, e.g., *Tāla (Narapuṣpa)*,
3. *vātapittaghnakaphodāsīna*, e.g., *Cañcu*

V. *kaphavātaghna varga*
1. *kaphavātaghna*, e.g., *Devadāru*,
2. *kaphavātaghnapittala*, e.g., *Varuṇa*,
3. *kaphavātaghnapittodāsīna*, e.g., *Vilva*,
4. *kaphavātaghnālpapittala*, e.g., *Śigruphala*

VI. *kaphapittaghna varga*,
1. *kaphapittaghna*, e.g., *Jambū*,
2. *kaphapittaghnavātakara*, e.g., *Karañja*,
3. *kaphapittaghnavatodāsīna*, e.g., *Tilaparṇī*,
4. *kaphapittaghnālpavātala*, e.g., *Taṇḍulīya*

VII. *doṣaghna varga*
1. *tridoṣaghna*, e.g., *Kāśmarī*

VIII. *doṣala varga*,
1. *vātala*, e.g., *Tila* (flower, greens),
2. *vātalālpapittakapha*, e.g., *Ruṇeyaka Phala*,

3. *pittala*, e.g., *Śamī* (fruit),
4. *śleṣmala*, e.g., *Mocarasa*,
5. *vātapittakara*, e.g., *Āmra* (tender fruits),
6. *vātapittakarakaphodāsīna*, e.g., *Kapittha* (unripe fruits),
7. *vātaśleṣmakara*, e.g., *Yaṣṭimadhu*,
8. *vātaśleṣmalālpapittakara*, e.g., *Yatuka* (*Keśaparṇi*),
9. *kaphapittakara*, e.g., *Āmra* (medium unripe),
10. *kaphapittakaravatodāsīna*, e.g., *Kusumbha Taila*,
11. *kaphapittakarālpavātala*, e.g., *Chatraka*,
12. *tridoṣala*, e.g., *Sarṣapa* (*Śāka*)

Wujastyk (2000) has analysed in detail the problems with combinatorics of flavour (*rasa*) and humour (*doṣa*) in Indian medical literature. He observes that the medical writers did not develop algorithms to work out their concept of combinatorics with mathematical precision.[20] The *Siddhamantra* is interesting in this context because Keśava is obviously not interested in mathematically deriving the combinatorics of the humours (*doṣa*). He follows an empirical approach and creates a classification based on actual observations of the properties of substances, which add up to 48 subgroups under eight broad groups. However, his son, Vopadeva does attempt to mathematically derive the combinatorics and ends up with a problematic list of 57 subgroups, which

[20]Wujastyk (2000: 479–95) observes, "The evidence above seems to show that the medical authors had understood the concept of combinatorics, but that they had not developed or were not aware of algorithms for producing results. These algorithmic methods seem only to have been used amongst the mathematicians from Varāhamihira, Mahāvīra, and Bhāskara onwards. Varāhamihira had an early form of algorithm, which appears rather clumsy to use in practice. Mahāvīra introduced (or at least was an early adopter of) a delightfully straightforward technique and was also the earliest author so far identified to use the medical problem of the flavours as an example of this algorithmic technique."

he fails to satisfactorily list and elaborate. Sharma (1977) does not throw further light on the logical inconsistencies of Vopadeva's listing, but his tabulation is very helpful in understanding Vopadeva's approach to deriving the combinatorics of the humours (*doṣa*). The combinatorics of the humours (*doṣa*) into 48 (57) subgroups under eight broader groups is a unique contribution of *Siddhamantra* in three ways. First, it is the concept of *udāsīna* that makes this classification unprecedented and different from what has been attempted in the earlier works. Secondly, the combinatorics of Caraka, Suśruta and Vāgbhaṭa are based on pathological derangement of the humours (*doṣa*) and Suśruta adds blood (*rakta*) along with the three humours (*doṣa*). On the other hand, for the first time, Keśava classifies medicinal substances on the basis of their pharmacological action on the *doṣa*s.

Reconciliation of contradictions amongst authorities

Keśava expresses concern that the views of celebrated authorities in the field of Ayurveda should contradict each other when it comes to the delineation of pharmacological properties. Taking the example of honey, Keśava points out that Caraka characterizes it as an aggravator of wind (*vāta*),[21] while Suśruta deems it to be a pacifier of wind (*vāta*).[22] On the other hand, Khāraṇādi does not specify it as either an aggravator of pacifier of wind (*vāta*). Vopadeva

[21]Properties of honey as described in the *Carakasaṃhitā sūtrasthāna* 27, v. 245 (Ācārya 1941: 167) are as follow: *vātalaṃ guru śītañ ca raktapittakaphāpaham| sandhātṛ cchedanaṃ rūkṣaṃ kaṣāyaṃ madhuraṃ madhu|*

[22]The properties of honey as described in the *Suśrutasaṃhitā sūtrasthāna*, 132 (Ācārya 1938: 207), are as follow: *madhu tu madhuraṃ kaṣāyānurasaṃ rūksaṃ śītām agnidīpanaṃ varṇyaṃ svaryaṃ laghu sukumāraṃ lekhanaṃ hṛdyaṃ vājīkaraṇaṃ sandhānaṃ ropaṇaṃ (saṃgrāhi) cakṣu-*

points out in his commentary that Keśava has reconciled such contradictions in case of honey and other substances like *vetrāgra, koradūṣa, paṭola* and *tālasasya*.[23]

Keśava's approach is reminiscent of Vāgbhaṭa's attempts to reconcile the contradictions between the *Carakasaṃhitā* and the *Suśrutasaṃhitā*. Indu (*fl. ca.* 1100–1150), in his *Śaśilekhā* commentary on the *Aṣṭāṅgasaṅgraha*, points out that the contradiction in delineating the properties of the water from rivers that flow out of the Himalayan ranges in the texts of Caraka and Suśruta have been reconciled by Vāgbhaṭa. According to Caraka, the waters flowing from the Himalayan ranges are wholesome and good for health.[24] However, according to Kṛṣṇātreya and Suśruta, they cause illnesses like growths in the neck and the like.[25] Vāgbhaṭa resolves this controversy by explaining that the water from the mountains that flow forcefully against the

---

ṣyaṃ prasādanaṃ sūkṣmamārgānusāri pittaśleṣmamedomehahikkāśvāsakāsātisāracchardītṛṣṇākṛmiviṣapraśamanaṃ hlādi tridoṣapraśamanaṃ ca|

[23]Vopadeva clarifies how the logic of resolving the controversies regarding the properties of honey can be applied to other drugs (Sharma 1977: section 2, p. 8): *tathā ca carakeṇa vetrāgraṃ vātaleṣu paṭhitam…|. khāraṇādinā tridoṣaghneṣu paṭhitam…| tad apy atra madhuvan nirṇītaṃ| ata eva suśrutena kaphapittaghnam evoktam|*

[24]In this verse, Caraka explains that the waters that are broken and dispersed by falling on stones and flowing from the Himalayan ranges are pure, wholesome and used by gods and sages (Ācārya 1941: 171): *nadyaḥ pāṣāṇavicchinnavikṣubdhābhihatodakāḥ| himavatprabhavāḥ pathyāḥ puṇyāḥ devarṣisevitāḥ|.*

[25]Suśruta says that the water from rivers originating in the Himalayas cause heart disease, swelling, diseases of head and swelling in the neck (Ācārya 1938: 213): *tatra sahyaprabhavāḥ kuṣṭhaṃ janayanti vindhyaprabhavāḥ kuṣṭhaṃ pāṇḍurogaṃ ca malayaprabhavāḥ kṛmīn māhendraprabhavāḥ ślīpadodarāṇi himavatprabhavāḥ hṛdrogaśvayathuśirorogaślīpadagalagaṇḍān prācyāvantyā aparāvantyāścārśāṃsyupajanayanti pāriyātraprabhavāḥ pathyāḥ balārogyakarāya iti|.*

rocks are wholesome for health while they are harmful when stagnant.[26]

Theoretical construct to facilitate reconciliation

What makes this classification unique, however, is the introduction of the novel concept termed *udāsīna* or 'neutral' to indicate a neutral effect on the humours (*doṣa*).[27] This means that the effects of substances on the *doṣa*s are evaluated in terms of whether they pacify, disturb or have no effect on the humours (*doṣa*).

In the example of honey, Keśava's contention is that it is wind-neutral (*vātodāsīna*), that is, inherently neutral with respect to wind (*vāta*). Because it is inherently neutral, it can behave as aggravator or pacifier of wind (*vāta*) depending on conditions like dosage, time factor, combination etc. By itself, pure honey can neither aggravate nor pacify wind (*vāta*), but when conditioned it can be an aggravator or pacifier of wind (*vāta*). Interpreted thus, the contradictions in the statements of Caraka and Suśruta get resolved and the silence of Khāraṇādi with regard to the action of honey on

---

[26]The commentator Indu explains in his commentary on *Aṣṭāṅgasaṅgraha* how Vāgbhaṭa has resolved the contradictory statements in the works of Caraka and Suśruta (Āṭhavale 1980: 4): *paratantravirodho yathā carakagranthena kṛṣṇātreyo viruddhaḥ, tathā carako himavatprabhavānām nadīnāṃ pathyatvam icchanti, kṛṣṇātreyasuśrutau tāsām eva galagaṇḍādikartṛtvaṃ, vāgbhaṭas tūpalasphāletyādinā virodhaṃ nivartayati – upalāsphālanakṣepavicchedaiḥ kheditodakāḥ, himavanmalayodbhutaḥ pathyāsta eva ca sthitāḥ, kṛmiślīpadahṛtkaṇṭhaśirorogān prakurvate|*

[27]Vopadeva explains the logic of the validity of the concept of *audāsīnya* (Sharma 1977: section 2, p. 7): *niṣpratibandha upādhivyāpāre vātalopahitasya madhuno vātalatve nyāyasiddhe vacanavaiyarthyam iti cen na, asiddhe hy audāsīnye nyāyapravṛttir iti iha tv asmad eva vacanān nyāyasahakṛtād audāsīnyasiddhiḥ|*

wind (*vāta*) can be put into perspective.[28]

Brevity in expressing a vast subject in a compact manner

Keśava claims that it is a matter of amazement only to the dull-witted that the determination of the pharmacological property of a substance not discussed in this work will not be found elsewhere. He means to say that the dull-witted might wonder how a work that is so brief can be so comprehensive and all-inclusive. In other words, the intelligent reader will be able to appreciate the skills of the author in composing this work.

The commentator Vopadeva remarks that it is impossible to capture the infinite range of medicinal substances within the scope of a book. But the *Siddhamantra* has extensively compiled information from all the available and authoritative sources of Ayurveda and in that respect becomes quite comprehensive and complete even when it is extremely concise.[29]

Snippets from the commentary of Vopadeva

Siddhamantra would lose much of its charm were it not for the learned commentary of Vopadeva. Being the son

---

[28]Vopadeva explains how the controversy surrounding the properties of honey can be resolved with the help of the concept of *audāsīnya* (Sharma 1977: section 2, p. 7): *tasmāc chuddham madhu vātodāsīnam ity abhihitaṃ, tattūpādhibhedādvāt alaṃ vātaghnañ cety ucitaṃ, upadhayaś ca mātrādayaḥ|*

[29]Vopadeva clarifies how this work is comprehensive in spite of being very brief (Sharma 1977: section 2, p. 66): *yady apy ānantyād dravyāṇi kārtsnyena vaktum aśakyāni tathāpi yāvanti prācīneṣu grantheṣu labdhāni tāvanti nirṇītānīty arthaḥ| atra viṣaye adhīmatām buddhivihīnānām citram katham īdṛśenātisamkṣiptena granthena tādṛg vistīrṇacarakādiśāstroktasamagradravyanirṇayaity anupapattigarbho vismayaḥ, na tu buddhimatām|*

of Keśava, Vopadeva has perhaps preserved the original thought process of the author and his interpretations are crucial in throwing light on some of the key verses, which by themselves would leave much to the imagination of the reader.

For instance, the verse that alludes to the contradiction between the views of Caraka, Suśruta and Khāraṇādi does not mention that the discussion is about honey. Vopadeva makes this explicit in his commentary.[30]

Keśava only mentions that he has resolved contradictions between the authorities. It is Vopadeva who gives an elaborate account of the methodology and the arguments with examples of how this is achieved by the author.

Keśava does not mention generic power (*prabhāva*) when he enumerates the factors that determine drug action. Vopadeva explains that *prabhāva* is not a property of the drug.[31]

Vopadeva's commentary is studded with succinct remarks and statements that are quite revelatory. In one context he mentions that the author considers three authorities as the most reliable amongst many others. Interestingly, these authorities form a triad that is not a familiar combination in the tradition of Ayurveda – Caraka, Suśruta and Khāraṇādi. Sharma takes it for granted that Caraka, Suśruta and Vāgbhaṭa form the triad referred to by Vopadeva and Keśava.[32] However, on a closer look, it is

[30]Vopadeva points out that Keśava is referring to honey in the particular verse (Sharma 1977: section 2, p. 6): *vātalam carako brute vātaghnam vaṣti suśrutaḥ, khāraṇādir vadaty anyo, ity ukter atra nirṇayaḥ – yathā madhu carakeṇa vātalam uktaṃ|*

[31]Sharma 1977: section 2, p. 3: *prabhāvasya tv asadhāraṇadravyalakṣanān atiriktalakṣanatvan na guṇatvam|*

[32]Sharma comments (1977: section 2, intro. p. 10), "While accepting the authority, the commentator accepts only three, Caraka, Suśruta and

quite obvious that the third authority is Khāraṇādi and not Vāgbhaṭa. In fact, Keśava refutes the views of Vāgbhaṭa in favor of Suśruta when they contradict each other.[33] But on a closer look, it is quite obvious that Vopadeva is commenting on the verse composed by Keśava that mentions Caraka, Suśruta and Khāraṇādi, by name, and not Vāgbhaṭa. Vopadeva justifies the authority of this triad on the grounds that their works are credible, complete, have an unbroken tradition and have been commented upon by eminent scholars in the field.[34]

It is interesting to note that Vopadeva underplays the authority of Vāgbhaṭa when he contradicts Suśruta in deciphering the pharmacological properties of palm grain (*talasasya*). According to Vāgbhaṭa, palm grain (*talasasya*) aggravates bile (*pitta*) and has a laxative liquid (*sāra*) action. On the other hand, Suśruta attributes to it the ability to pacify bile (*pitta*) and mentions that it is heavy to digest. Vopadeva explains that Vāgbhaṭa has misread the word *rasa* "taste" as *sāra* "liquid" and *pittahṛd* "bile-heart" as *pittakṛt* "bile-producing," and thus wrongly interpreted its pharmacological properties. He further quotes Caraka and Khāraṇādi in support of Suśruta and concludes that Keśava has characterized palm grain (*talasasya*) as a pacifier of wind (*vāta*) and bile (*pitta*) and aggravator of phlegm (*kapha*).[35]

Vāgbhaṭa because they are complete, traditionally unbroken and commented on by scholars."

[33]See Sharma 1977: section 2, p. 10.

[34]Vopadeva spells out the criteria for credibility of the authorities accepted by Keśava as follows (Sharma 1977: section 2, p. 10): *carakādīnāṃ trayāṇām evopādānaṃ, tatpraṇītatantrāṇāṃ pramāṇatvāt, sampūrṇatvād avicchinnasampradāyatvād abhiyuktair vyākhyātatvāc ca|*

[35]Vopadeva explains why the view of Vāgbhaṭa is not acceptable when compared with that of Suśruta (Sharma 1977: section 2, p. 10): *ata eva tad-*

Vopadeva's commentary is replete with quotations from various authorities in the field of Ayurveda, many of whose works have been lost subsequently. His commentary is also very valuable in fixing the identities of the medicinal and food substances mentioned by Keśava.

Discussion

Keṣava stands out in the tradition of Ayurveda for his original thinking, critical approach, innovative ideas and practical outlook. Being an accomplished clinician himself, Keśava realized the importance of precision devoid of ambiguities in deciphering and understanding the pharmacological properties of medicinal substances. Though critical, he is also very respectful of the authorities and the tradition of Ayurveda. He employs his intellectual prowess to authenticate the traditional teachings of Ayurveda with the help of new theoretical constructs, clever arguments and new classifications. And the novelty of his innovative ideas gets subsumed in the service of those authorities whom he selects as the most credible.

The commentary of Vopadeva reveals the aggressive attitude of Keśava in refuting the views of many authorities in the process of justifying his own interpretations. But Keśava expresses equal vehemence when it comes to defending and reconciling the views of those whom he considers to be the ultimate authorities on the subject.

---

viruddhānām anyeṣām aprāmāṇyam eva| yathā phalaṃ tu pittalaṃ tālaṃ saram iti vāgbhaṭavākyasya phalaṃ svādu rase teṣāṃ tālajaṃ guru pittahṛd iti suśrutavākyavirodhāt...kiñ ca rasam ity atra saram iti, hṛd ity atra kṛd ity anyathā gṛhītaṃ suśrutavākyam evātra mūlaṃ sambhāvyate|

Conclusion

The *Siddhamantra* of Keśava is an important work that has been neglected by scholars and practitioners of Ayurveda in contemporary times. There is no doubt that this work has historical importance for the novel ideas and approaches that it has brought forth in the field of Ayurvedic pharmacology. However, it has to be pointed out that Keśava was not a mere theoretician and he was not building up his arguments merely on the basis of textual analysis. As Vopadeva has pointed out, his father recorded the properties of the drugs accurately, as observed by himself, and did not forcefully classify them into predetermined groups.[36] The uniqueness of *Siddhamantra* rests on the fact that its author was a clinician of no mean order and his clinical experiences contributed significantly in helping him arrive at decisive insights on the pharmacological properties of controversial medicinal substances. The *Siddhamantra* is thus the "hymn of success," exemplifying a rigorous approach to corroborate clinical experience with textual analysis in arriving at a deeper understanding of the classical writings of Ayurveda.

Further reading

Ācārya, Yādavaśarman Trivikrama (ed.) 1938. *Suśrutasaṃhitā, Suśrutena viracitā, VaidyavaraśrīḌalhaṇācāryaviracitayā Nibandhasaṃgrahākhyavyākhyayā samullasitā, Ācāryopāhvena Trivikramātmajena Yādavaśarmaṇā saṃśodhitā.* Mumbayyāṃ: Nirṇayasāgara Mudrāyantrālaye, 3rd edn. Consulted in the 1994 reprint (Varanasi: Chaukhambha Surabharati).

[36]Vopadeva remarks that the properties of substances have been documented exactly as they have been observed (Sharma 1977: section 2, p. 12): *yatra dravye yo dṛṣṭaḥ sa tatrokta eva| yathā vātaghnī pittalā cālpakaphā cāpy akṣikī suretyādi|*

— 1941. *Maharṣiṇā Punarvasunopadiṣṭā, tacchiṣyeṇāgniveśena praṇītā, CarakaDṛḍhabalābhyāṃ pratisaṃskṛtā Carakasaṃhitā, śrīCakrapāṇidattaviracitayā āyurvedadīpikāvyākhyayā saṃvalitā.* Mumbayyāṃ: Nirṇayasāgara Mudrāyantrālaye, 3rd edn. Consulted in the 2002 reprint (Varanasi: Chaukhambha Surabharati).

Āṭhavale, Anaṃta Dāmodara (ed.) 1980. *Aṣṭāṅgasaṅgrahaḥ. ŚrīmadVṛddhavāgbhaṭaviracitaḥ Induvyākhyāsahitaḥ.* Puṇe: Maheśa Anaṃta Āṭhavale, Śrīmad Ātreya Prakāśanam.

Bhaṭṭācārya, Tārānātha Tarkavācaspati 1969–1970. *Vācaspatyam, Bṛhat saṃskṛtābhidhānam = Vachaspatyam (a comprehensive Sanskrit dictionary)*, vol. 94 of *Caukhambā Saṃskṛta granthamālā.* Varanasi: Chowkhamba Sanskrit Series Office. 6v.

Kuṃṭe, Ananta Moreśvara, Kṛṣṇaśāstrī Rāmacandra Navare, and Hariśāstrī Parādkar (eds.) 1902. *Aṣṭāṅgahṛdayam, śrīmadVāgbhaṭaviracitam, sūtra-śārīra-nidāna-cikitsā-kalpa-uttarasthānavibhaktam śrīmadAruṇadattapraṇītayā sarvāṃgasuṃdaryākhyayā vyākhyayā samalaṃkṛtam*, vol. 3 of *Kṛṣṇadāsa Āyurveda Sīrīja.* Muṃbayyām: Nirṇayasāgara Press. Cited from the Varanasi: Chaukhambha Surabharati, 1994 reprint.

Meulenbeld, Gerrit Jan 1999–2002. *A History of Indian Medical Literature*, vol. XV of *Groningen Oriental Studies.* Groningen: E. Forsten. 5v.

— 2001. "Reflections on the Basic Concepts of Indian Pharmacology." In Gerrit Jan Meulenbeld and Dominik Wujastyk (eds.), *Studies on Indian Medical History*, vol. 5 of *Indian Medical Tradition*, pp. 1–17. Delhi: Motilal Banarsidass, 2nd edn. First edition Groningen, 1987.

Monier-Williams, Monier, E. Leumann, and C. Cappeller 1899. *A Sanskrit–English Dictionary Etymologically and Philologically Arranged, New Edition.* Oxford: Clarendon

Press. 1970 reprint.

Pade, Śaṅkara Dājīśāstrī and Śrī Bhālacandra (eds.) 1898. *Āyurvedasaṃgraha [including the Siddhamantra of Keśava]*. Bombay: Jñānasāgara Press.

Sharma, Priya Vrat (ed.) 1977. *Hṛdayadīpakanighaṇṭu Siddhamantraprakāśaś ca = Vopadeva's Hṛdayadīpaka nighaṇṭu and Siddhamantra of Vaidyācārya Keśava, with prakāśa commentary of Vopadeva*, vol. 1 of *Caukhambā āyurveda granthamālā*. Varanasi: Chaukhambha Amarabharati Prakashan.

Wujastyk, Dominik 2000. "The Combinatorics of Tastes and Humours in Classical Indian Medicine and Mathematics." *Journal of Indian Philosophy*, **28**, 479–95.

Index

Colophon

This book is typeset in the TEX Gyre Pagella typefaces, with old-style numerals and British English hyphenation.

The TEX Gyre family of fonts is rich in typographic extensions and accented characters and was created by Bogusław Jackowski, Janusz M. Nowacki and Piotr Strzelczyk for the Polish TEX Users Group on the basis of the URW Palladio L kindly released by URW++ Design and Development Inc. under the Gnu Font License.

TeX Gyre Pagella looks back to the renowned Palatino font designed by Hermann Zapf in the 1940's for the Stempel type foundry.

The typesetting tools were TEXLive 2012, XeLaTeX and TEXStudio, all running on GNU/Linux (Ubuntu 12.10).